P9-EJY-964

AROMATHERAPY
for Sensual Living

AROMATHERAPY
for Sensual Living

Essential Oils for the Ecstatic Soul

Elana Millman

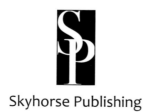

Skyhorse Publishing

Visit our website at www.skyhorsepublishing.com.

10 9 8 7 6 5 4 3 2 1

Library of Congress Cataloging-in-Publication Data is available on file.

Cover design by Erin Seaward Hiatt

Cover photo credit William Praniski

Print ISBN: 978-1-63220-336-6

Ebook ISBN: 978-1-63220-893-4

Printed in China

To the Great Mystery,

And my mother and father.

Eternally grateful.

‡

Photography by William Praniski

A Note to the Reader

Table of Contents

Acknowledgments

I am humbled by all those who have helped and contributed to the creation of *Aromatherapy for Sensual Living*. Sam Hiyate at the Right Factory, thank you for everything. You have a special place in my heart. Alex Hess at Skyhorse Publishing, for your work and vision. William Praniski, my amazingly talented rockstar photographer, for gorgeously bringing the visual component to life. Camila Derisé, my massage model in the jungle. Richard Sharp, it's pure joy to work and conspire with you. Liz Freud, Ashley Hain, Nicole Angela, Liliana Aldana Garcia, your beauty serves as constant inspiration throughout these pages. Nadine Artemis of Living Libations, my aroma mentor and sister friend, deepest gratitude and love forever. Sandra Bialystok and Andrea Aster, deep appreciation for your editorial feedback and being brilliant, exceptional women. My parents, Dorothy and Larry Millman, I am humbly grateful for your love and encouragement. Words cannot express. The rest of my family: Shawna, Leah, Sam, Violet and Auzine. Ajay Singh, my love for you is infinite. And to other important people who have generously contributed: Tatyanna Wilkinson, Owen James, Judith Marcelo, Sonia Palhares de Alverga, Roger Lewis, Janice Parsons, Aysha Parsons, Wayne Godfrey, Eddie Faria, Tara Menansky, Liz Riddell, Johanna Koeslag, Barbara Clark, Amanda Nabes, Cina Schmidt-Hansen, David Wolfe, Groove Das, Cindy Filler, Nakky Ottaway, Chris Savidge, Robyn Harrison for kitchen pick-up photography, Mo Bot, Alex Gillott, Brandon Fisher, Jen Wilson, Lori Myles, Carla Kearns, Rio de Janeiro, Brazil, and finally, to my dear, sweet essential oil friends, thank you for revealing your magic and beauty to me. Viva!

Introduction

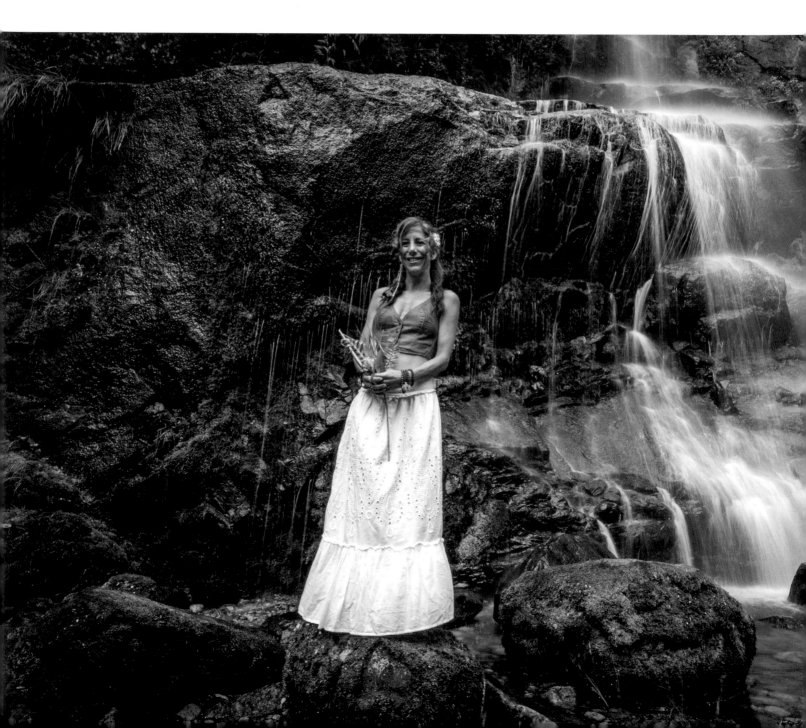

Aromatherapy has infiltrated our world. Many people have a bottle of lavender, peppermint, or even oregano tucked away for an emergency bout of insomnia or nausea, or to conquer a cold or flu. Through positive experimentation, people have come to understand that essential oils can be used not only to make a room smell beautiful, but for medicinal purposes too.

As such, aromatherapy is quickly becoming a staple for those who want to empower their own health and healing in harmonious vibration with the best of nature. Most people don't yet know the depth and breadth to which essential oils can heal and help; that's where I come in!

In *Aromatherapy for Sensual Living,* you will learn how to authentically imbibe essential oils every day, in every way, for every part of your life and love. You will discover the benefits of an ancient healing modality, and most importantly, you will ignite your essential juju juice — infinitely amplified and gloriously revealed.

Many of us are disconnected from the natural world. We feel more comfortable in the confines of a grey, concrete city than barefoot and wild, frolicking through the forest. We eat packaged, processed foods but are hesitant to eat weeds from our gardens, fearful of the poisons that may lurk. We slather ourselves with sun-blocking chemicals rather than embrace the rich hormonal cascade that can only be achieved by the sun's elegant rays. We're more inclined to hand over our power to doctors rather than use the time-tested guidance of our mothers and grandmothers.

Aromatherapy is the answer to this disconnection. However, aromatherapy is so much more than a candy-coated cure-all achieved by simply placing a few drops on a tissue or in an oil burner to get the promised relaxing or stimulating effect.

I use essential oils every day and in every way, from stimulating my love life to healing a broken heart, to brushing my teeth, to treating a wound and even flavoring my food. They provide a healthy dose of positivity everywhere I go!

This book takes aromatherapy out of the classroom and into the kitchen, home spa, and bedroom. You are invited to get down and go deep with power of the flowers. My goal is to demystify the mysterious and somewhat shadowy world of aromatherapy and make it easy, fun, and accessible so you will confidently use these precious libations as part of your regular practice.

Some books can be overly cautious with application guidelines and recommend doses that aren't strong enough do the trick. In doing so, they negate the expansive, exquisite healing powers of essential oils and turn them into trivial, prosaic mood-enhancers. In my world, there's a place for potency! In certain cases, I've administered essential oils every minute — undiluted and internally — until I corrected an imbalance. Other times, a single diluted drop heals within seconds. I trust them, use them and have never been let down by my essential oil friends. For me, there is no greater joy than inhaling a single drop of oil to feel entirely at ease and in perfect communion with the natural world.

As you develop your own relationship with these precious aromatics, you may have a different understanding of the individual properties than what I describe. That's perfect. For some, immortelle smells like a wild kaleidoscope of raw sensuality. To others, it smells like a pair of overripe gym socks. Trust your nose is guiding you to the perfect perfume and perfect partner. Your nose always knows.

Aromatherapy for Sensual Living encourages the reader to include essential oils to boost smoothies, enhance bath time, improve water flavor, deepen massage, compresses, and inhalations, treat the chakras, and increase sexual confidence. Essential oils are outstanding implements that impart enormous mental, physical, and spiritual benefits with surprising simplicity and potent results. My hope is that you will experiment to deepen your knowledge of the plant kingdom in an effortless, deeply sensuous, and enjoyable way.

I invite you to drink in the divine nectar of aromatic love and let it penetrate you in the deepest, most profound ways. Trust that the oils are working side-by-side to heal, regenerate, and teach you. The more you use them, the more they'll reveal their secrets to you. With even minimal skill, essential oils will easily and dramatically enhance your well being. Even after twenty years, I'm still humbled by the innate wisdom and lavish beauty that they bring to every aspect of my life.

And just like that, the petals part their lips and the flower begins to bloom.

– Elana Millman

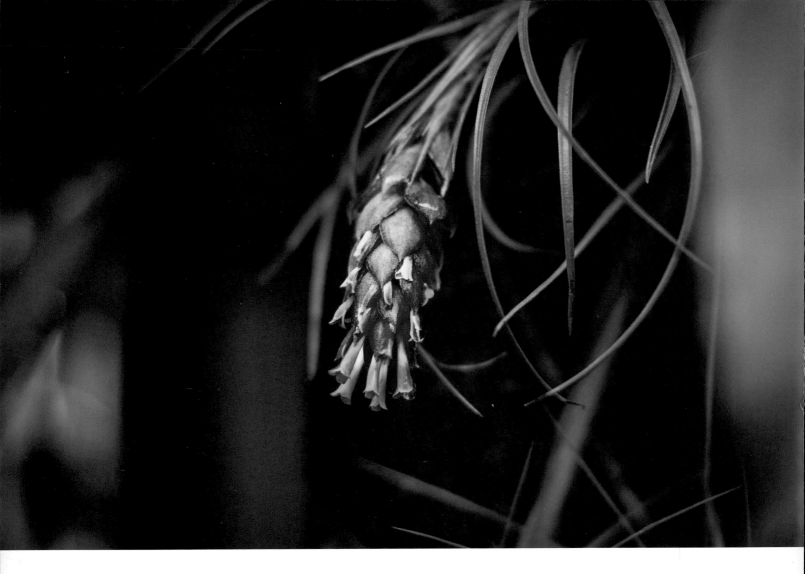

Sensuality and Our Senses

What is sensuality?

Sensuality relates to how we can move, shake, and beguile our (desired) beloved into a deeper sense of communion. It's a well-timed wink, the hug of cashmere on subtle curves, or the undulation of hips on a dance floor. It's salacious confidence seen in the way we hold ourselves in our bodies and in our lives.

Raw sensuality is not something that should be easily overlooked. For some, however, it's taboo or culturally inappropriate to express their divinely sensual feminine nature. I encourage you to buck the system and be sensual regardless of your age, culture, or body size. Explore your inner sensual strength (your wild woman power) so you walk with unshakable poise and an effortless glide in your stride. It's your sexy Shakti power waiting to be unleashed and unharnessed.

Another way to understand sensuality has nothing to do with titillating times. *Sensual Living* is being in the present moment, appreciating all the curious and astounding beauty that surrounds us. Sensuality is the ability to achieve pleasure through all of our senses simultaneously — right here, right now.

Look around your immediate environment, listen to the sounds around you, touch the clothes you're wearing, and

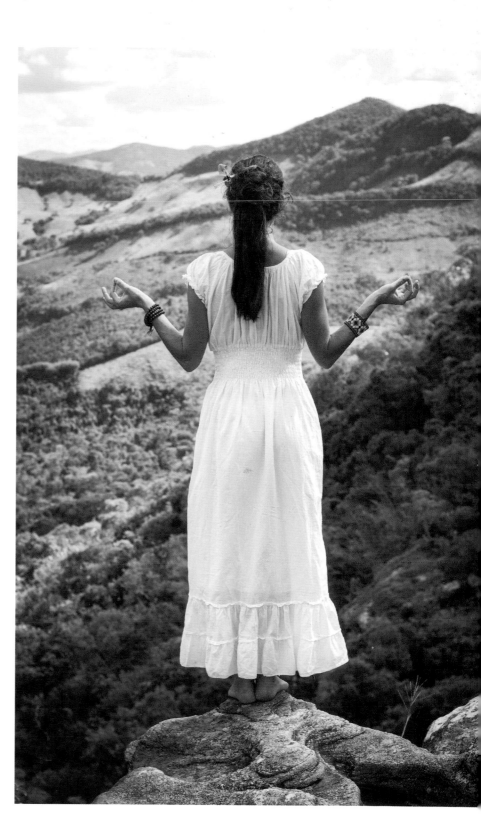

deeply inhale your skin. In doing so, you instantaneously become present and awake. It's by engaging our senses that we get closer to divine life force energy and are able to rest in the place of gratitude, peace, and love. Sensuality resides in our ability to breathe, be open, and receive. This awareness quiets our busy minds and lets our sympathetic nervous system relax and unwind. It's an important practice and one that only improves other facets of life, especially the horizontal ones.

Essential oils have the mysterious ability to awaken our natural and effervescent sensuality. They're divine treasures that:

- lift our spirits and infuse us with good, positive, confident feelings

- bring us into the present moment

- heal our mind, body, and spirit on the deepest levels

Pure perfume and divine spirit perform the same function.

Essential oils present a way to physically hold and utilize the gifts of the great spirit in our very own hands. We get to play with, rub on, and consume splendid divine power to make our lives and health better. It's astoundingly powerful and utterly humbling. By working with essential oils, we harness concentrated plant power and are able to commune deeply at the highest realms.

Essential *Oil Eroticism*

I've spent many wonderful days (and nights) "researching" different ways to employ essential oils to deepen sensual play and erotic provocation. I discovered that essential oils can greatly intensify the connection and charisma between you and your lover. This isn't just a hopeful desire, but pulsating reality. Sensual aromatherapy is powerful stuff. When you use essential oils for sensual play, you change brain chemistry by bypassing the blood-brain barrier and moving directly into the seat of desire through the hypothalamus and limbic brain — the oldest part of our brains. It's the place of "I want you and there's nothing I won't do to have you and have you now!" The easiest methods of application are in a room spray, on a drop of honey, or a discreet mist on the neck. But that's only the beginning.

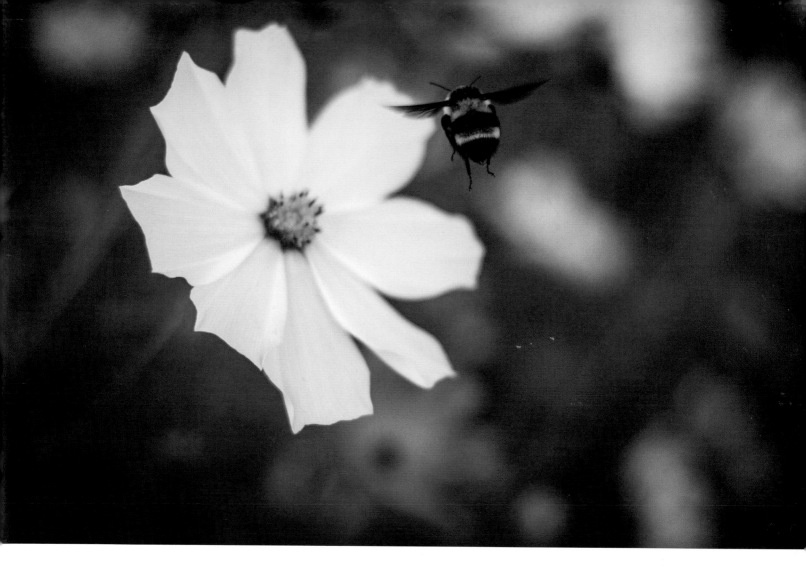

I get excited thinking about how to create personalized smell-scapes by using my knowledge of essential oils and their properties. I curate a space and the emotions I want to evoke by using specific essential oils in the right concentrations. It's total witchy magic.

Through the years, I've used this wisdom to get my desired result. Sometimes it led to smoldering delights and other times it was just a plain bad idea.

Some lovers are simply not ready for a drop of expensive rose otto or a luscious whiff of immortelle. For some with compromised immune systems or toxicity due to hard living, illness, or high stress, essential oils can be aggravating rather than enlivening. How one reacts to essential oils is a wonderful barometer of health and vitality. Beautiful flower, I ask that you choose a suitor who is tickled by aroma love.

Explain how you plan to tempt and tease your lover with aromatic libations. People intrinsically understand that there's a potent connection between smell and sex (most likely because of the link to our ancient limbic brains). All men whom I've encountered are just a little bit curious as to how to employ essential oils to make intimacy even hotter. Once you have their agreement and some basic principles to follow, you'll have them eating out of the palm of your hand — or other places, you lucky sprite.

The sexiest part of the body for me is the mind; full of creativity, ingenuity, and sparkle. We can use our minds and our focused intention to heighten the connection with our love. Take a moment to refine your intention before lovemaking. Is it simply getting your rocks off, or connecting to the divine force of creation, or simply getting it done to get to sleep? Essential oils are perfect for whatever it is you're looking to achieve.

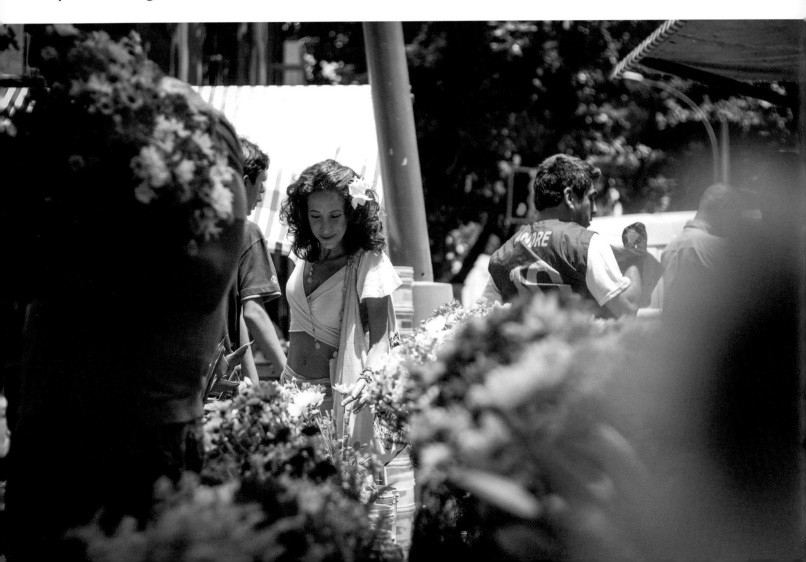

Aromatherapy in lovemaking inspires us to slow down and enjoy the process of creation with our beloved. It takes time to smell, create, drop, and blend together. Slowness and anticipation of what's to come is part of the fun. Savor the moment or, with luck, hours. Feel the power of the flowers to help guide you as to how many drops to use and which method is most appropriate to make it a tingly, exalted experience. And even if you drop one more than you intended, trust that the flowers are working with you and it's perfect too.

There's so much room for experimentation and play with aromatic sensuality. There's no need to get bored with the same-old-same-old when you have an abundance of oils and methods to choose. By using a variety of oils, you can create entirely different opportunities and responses. You're only limited by your own creativity, and I'm here to spark your imagination.

Sexy *Blending Practices for Men*

Not surprisingly, most men are quite receptive to the use of essential oils on their intimate members — especially if it leads to better and more passionate nights. Of course, there are some oils that should never be used on delicate skin, including cassia bark, cinnamon, black pepper, peppermint, clove, and ginger. There are several blends that work really well on a roused man-rod. Most men prefer the smells of trees, roots, resins, and leaves over flowers and many euphorics, though I've met men who simply adore the sweet smells of carnation, geranium, and ylang ylang.

One of my favorite combinations exclusively for men is blending the essential oils of 30 percent sandalwood, 20 percent cypress, 25 percent blood orange and 25 percent white cedar in two tablespoons of coconut oil, honey, or jojoba. I've given this blend to many female clients with frigid or stressed-out partners. It works beautifully to enhance sexy time, evoke their virile vigor, and is utterly spine-tingling.

Sandalwood is used because it's a euphoric. It's mellow, masculine, and romantic. Sandalwood both relaxes and stimulates in all the right ways. I haven't met a man that doesn't have a visceral positive response to this oil. That's just about the perfect place to invite aromatic lovemaking for your man.

Cypress moves energy and blood, and breaks up stagnation. It helps to activate the blend and bring dynamism, stamina, and vitality to your man and his sexual practices. Cypress is fresh, clean, and inviting. It will help him stay "at attention" to be able to play with you all night long.

Blood orange brings levity and playfulness to the blend, making sex fun and light-hearted. There's no need to just focus on the orgasmic prize. This oil keeps the practice (and blend) joyful rather than so heady it hurts. Blood orange will also relax him.

White cedar is pure masculine, loin-quivering juju juice. I've never smelled it on a man and didn't want to get a little closer and nuzzle up to his neck. It makes me purr. White cedar clears energy, moves stagnation, and improves physical function.

These oils combined together make for a very pleasant and erotic blend. The other benefit of this blend is that all the oils are steam-distilled. This means that you're welcome, in fact encouraged, to rub it on his body and then lick it off — special, sensitive parts included, and deeply appreciated.

Perfume's *Attraction*

Perfume has a long connection with flirtation, seduction, and amore. Perfume is a whisper, a come hither finger, and an invitation to close the door to make moving magic. To fully appreciate the toe-curling effect, perfume needs to be appreciated on warm skin, up close and personal, and with just enough to inform rather than overpower. It can linger for days on a lover's forgotten piece of clothing, and smelling it can recall rapture and quivering excitement in our minds and bodies. Smell is powerful stuff.

Sadly, for a lot of people, perfume has a negative connotation. Commercial perfume is synthetic, often toxic, hence the reason why so many people have allergic reactions to it. It's a gross perversion of what's available to the eager aroma enthusiast. Why bother with commercial substitutes when you can have authentic, natural-from-the-earth, artesian essential oils at your fingertips? Our bodies rebel against the chemical soup that we live in and are craving, even suffering for what's authentic, whole,

aromatherapy for sensual living *sensuality and our senses*

unadulterated, and sensuous. Those aromatic dish detergents, wall plug-ins, and scented candles are a gross and artificial deviation of what's real and available for us to use.

In this book, I use the terms perfume, essential oils, and aromatherapy interchangeably to talk about the pure, genuine aromas.

Pure perfume is unadulterated sensuality and a fast track to pulsating health. Our bodies intrinsically know and understand authentic aroma and respond accordingly, often with the desire for more. Up until recently, humans lived harmoniously in the forest and were in constant communication with the natural world and all who inhabit it every day, all the time. Because humans and plants have simultaneously evolved, adapted, and benefited from each other, we respond viscerally to scent as a way to navigate our world, find food, or even detect a suitable mate.

Pure perfume is created from pure essential oils from barks, roots, resins, flowers, seeds, fruit skins, grasses, shrubs, needles, wood, twigs, and leaves, and use water, alcohol, waxes, or fats as a base. Essential oils are the *amrita* or vital nectar of the plant. They're also the soul and immune system and a rather clever way to attract insects for pollination.

Essential oils are amazingly supportive to our health and vitality. All essential oils are antibacterial, antiviral, antifungal, antibiotic, and antiseptic. I call them the "anti-anti's" because they do so much to help us and, at the same time, get rid of the bad stuff. Pure perfumes are infinitely intelligent and only pursue and destroy what's harmful to us. They know the difference because flowers and humans have commingled with each other for millennia. Essential oils fortify our immune, circulatory, digestive, reproductive, respiratory, nervous, musculoskeletal, and skin systems. In aromatherapy, we use the precious nectar that the plants use to heal themselves. It's pure magic.

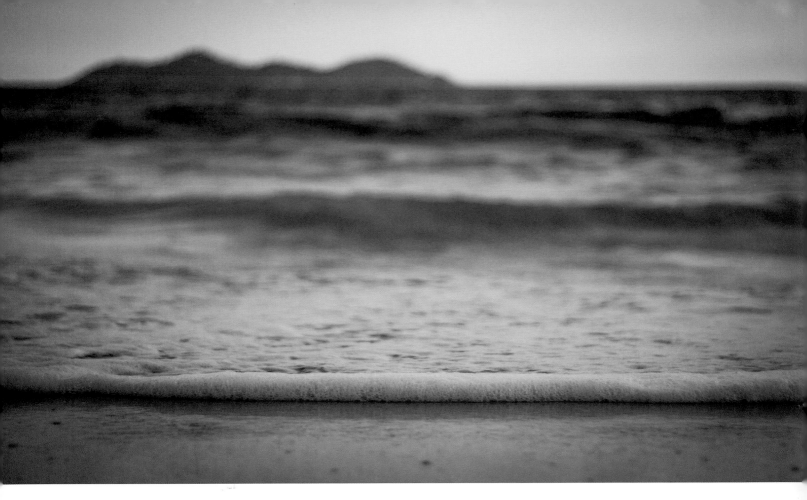

A Perfumed Ride Through History

History *of Perfume*

Societies have been distilling plants for beauty, perfume, and medicine for more than 5,000 years. Sacred herbs and medicines were traded and exchanged along trade routes to create, distill, and use as an ancient aroma apothecary. There are documents of perfume production in ancient Egypt,

Persia, China, India, and Japan. In fact, pots have been found at 5,500-year-old Sumerian sites which are believed to have been used for primitive extraction of essential oils. Our desire to imbibe the natural world is ancient, inherent, and lasting.

The Egyptians coined the term perfume from the Latin "per fumum," meaning through smoke. Smoke, in the form of incense and unguents, douses the recipient in aromas. There's evidence of cedarwood, frankincense, saffron, myrrh, cardamom, cinnamon, cassia, cypress, and calamus used in Egyptian ritual incense or as embalming agents. Rather morbidly, ancient Egyptian mummies were sometimes sold and distilled in the seventeenth century to be used as medicines themselves. Even after thousands of years, the mummies were still impregnated with the residue of potent medicinal aromatics.

Hippocrates, the father of Western medicine, wrote "a perfumed bath and a scented massage every day is the way to good health." I completely agree.

Persians came to the forefront of perfume creation around the tenth century by gathering information from Europe, India, and China. Avicenna, a poet and physician, developed and perfected the steam distillation method with a coiled cooling rod. That same method is used today.

Europe was struck down by the plague in the fourteenth century. Frankincense was burned to rid the streets of the smell of rotting flesh, give people their last rites, and try to contain the disease. A small band of grave robbers used aromatic vinegar made of clove, lemon, cinnamon, eucalyptus, and rosemary to fortify their health during looting quests. When caught, the grave robbers revealed that they were spice traders who knew herbal secrets, and they received lighter sentences in exchange for their potent wisdom. Their blend is still being used today by many aroma houses to cure illness and strengthen immunity. Perfumers and distillers at the time had to be protected by guards because the perfumers were immune to the disease (because of the antiseptic nature of essential oils), thus triggering suspicion that they were either holy, ascended beings, or workers of the devil.

By the sixteenth century, production of essential oils was widespread and many manor homes in England and Europe had still rooms devoted to the production of flower waters and essential oils. From the Middle Ages to the end of the eighteenth century, bathing was prohibited by the church except at birth and death. As such, people generously perfumed themselves to negate a lifetime of personal stink and utilize (without their full understanding) the antibacterial, antiseptic qualities inherent to all essential oils.

Perfume was elevated to a high art in the seventeenth century. Wealthy women had their personal jewelers create ornate boxes and jars to store their precious liquids. At that time, perfumed gloves were fashionable, as were poisons that were sometimes mixed with perfumes for some unlucky ladies.

Louis XIV's palace came to be known as "the perfumed court" in the eighteenth century. King Louis, known for his love of luxury and indulgence, demanded a different perfume for his apartment every day. Throughout the palace, several bowls were placed with flower petals to sweeten the air. Perfume was sprayed on to furniture, fans, and clothing. Even the water fountains were scented with perfume at Versailles. However, at the end of Louis XIV's life, any perfume, with the exception of neroli, would trigger violent migraines.

Perfume was in high demand across Europe at this time. To keep up, vast aromatic flower fields were planted in Grasse, France, that are still producing quality, potent essential oils today.

Authentic natural perfume sadly fell out of fashion in the nineteenth century as chemicals were created to produce variations or adulterations of the natural world. The inherent medicinal properties of natural essential oils were mostly lost, and a new and very lucrative synthetic fragrance market was born. The power and potency of aromatherapy was diminished for about 100 years.

True aromatherapy was rediscovered in the 1920s by French chemist Gatte-Fosse who, while researching essential oils, burned his hand very badly. Instinctively, he put his hand into a vat of lavender oil. The pain was immediately reduced and he healed quickly and without scarring. Gatte-Fosse reinvented modern aromatherapy and laid the groundwork for a renewed interest in natural, aromatic health and beauty.

Through trial and error, we've found that the blood of plants, the spirit of leaves, and the soul of flowers can be used for our beauty, perfume, and medicine. It's a union and communion of deep knowing, unlimited expansion, and whole-hearted appreciation. Essential oils can be used in every imaginable way. The aromatic path is one of love and self-healing. Love it all.

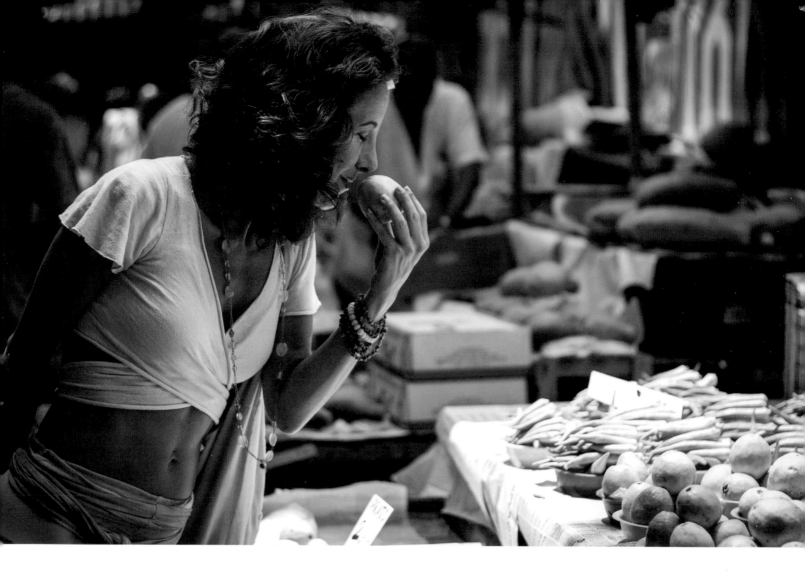

How to Smell: The Nose Knows

Sniff *Out the Truth*

Our ancient noses were far more adept at smelling than now. Sadly, our incredible, informative sense of smell has been diminished in our modern convenient, "antibacterial" world. Smell can invoke strong emotions and memories by being intimately connected to the limbic or reptilian brain (the oldest part of our brains). We can instantly and viscerally be transported back to a moment in time with a simple whiff of a familiar aroma. The limbic system is responsible for hormone production, memory, desire, and emotion. I invite you to use it rather than lose it; feast on flowers to improve your power of smell.

Aromatic *Discernment*

There are a lot of bad essential oils, fragrances, and perfume oils out there. A lot of "pure" essential oils are synthetic, adulterated, folded, fractionated, or extracted to have only a portion of their medicinal and aromatic components. The result is many synthetic or partially synthetic oils that are often easier and cheaper to produce. The smells are flat rather than fragrant. So how do you know if you have an authentic, awesomely alive, healing, and sensual quality oil? Smell it.

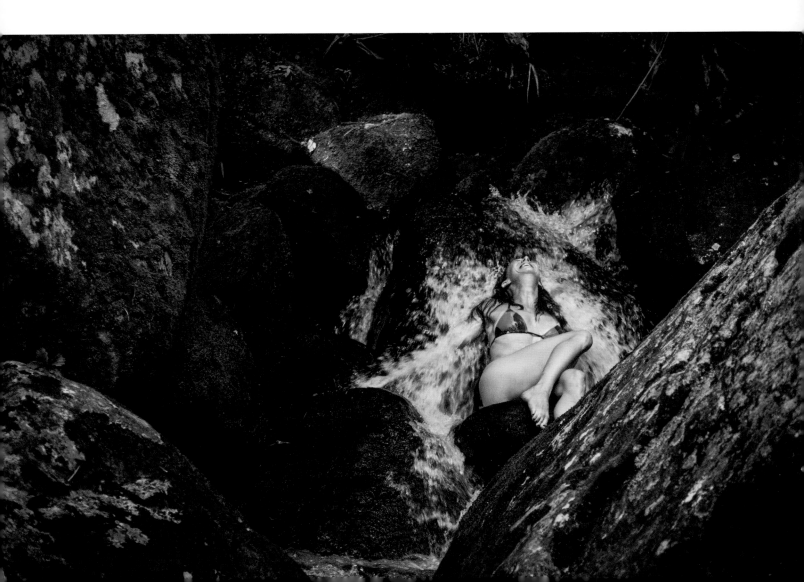

We're intelligent creatures. Our noses instantly know if something is whole, organic, and user-friendly much like we know instantly if there is subtle steamy chemistry between two people.

Simply smell deeply. Let the aroma fill you up. Track where the aroma goes in your body. If you take in the aroma and you feel relaxed, find yourself nodding yes, or break into an instant smile, you can rest assured that you've found the good stuff. Alternatively, if your body recoils in any way, it's not an authentic, medicinal-quality essential oil. If you find that your nose turns up even a little bit, you can bet that there are nasty synthetics or adulterations involved. If you get a little nauseous, dizzy, aggravated, anxious, or repulsed, put it down and try another brand.

There is one caveat, however. When you smell, you're actively taking in the aromatic and medicinal aspects of the plant. Sometimes you may sneeze, cough, or even turn away. Your body could be having a healing response. That's a good thing. Essential oils, in addition to being potent powerhouses of raw sensuality, are also incredibly medicinal.

Discernment, in aromatherapy and in love, is the key. Practice smelling and you'll soon be able to differentiate between authentic, real-to-the-feel essential oils and scented (horrendous) perfume products.

There are several different ways to take in an aroma. If you smell something unfamiliar and potentially synthetic, take a quick, short whiff through the nose. If it passes the body repulsion test, take a long and slow deep breath through your nose. Hold it for a moment to allow the scent molecules to enter into the body and bypass the blood-brain barrier. Exhale slowly. Follow with a series of short, rhythmic breaths into the nose like how a dog smells when it's searching for a buried bone. Inhale quickly and as many times as you can without feeling strained. Hold for a moment and release. Finally, take another long and slow deep breath in through the nose.

You might notice that the aroma changes slightly. Try using different methods of breathing, such as alternative nostril breathing, to receive the fullness of the aroma and to simply stop and smell the flowers.

Feast exclusively on quality aromatherapy to experience the true magnitude of essential oils (from companies like www.purfrequency.com). It's a wonderful activity to do with your love friend. Together you can imbibe essential oils and transcend space and time. It's pretty hot.

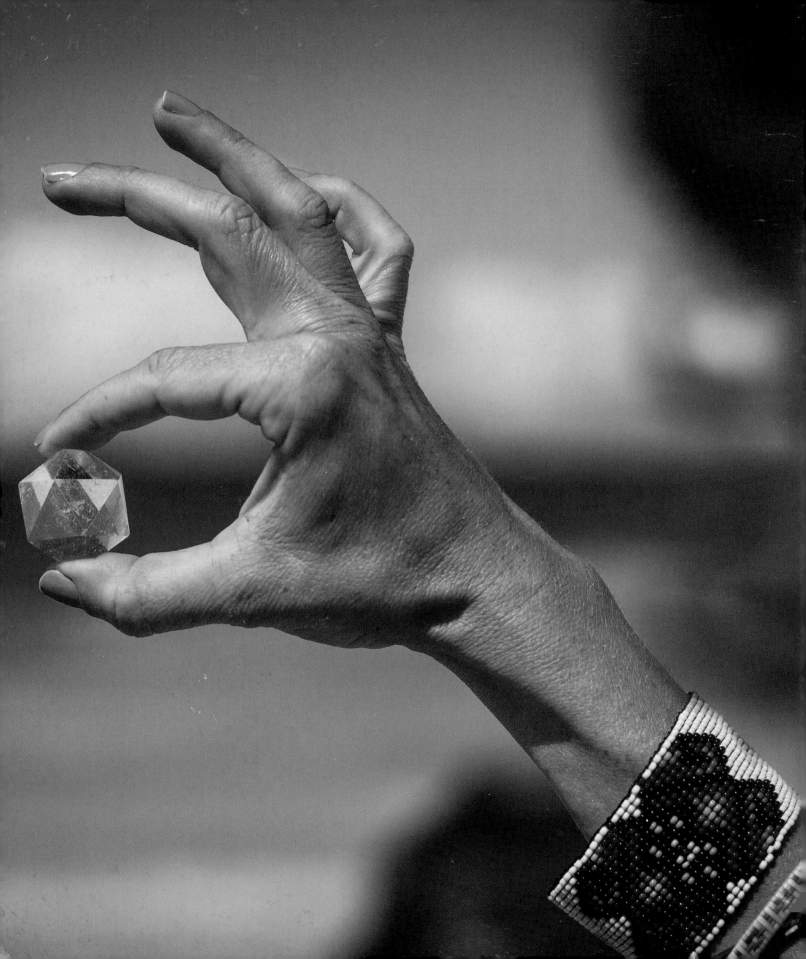

Deepening *Sensuality: Tangerine Temptation*

Hold a tangerine and observe its color, fragrance, shape, and texture. Spot any markings, indentations, or discolorations on the skin by using your eyes to truly take it in. Take note of the weight in your hand. Feel its plumpness.

Start to slowly peel the tangerine while noting the individual white threads inside. As you peel it, observe the zest: this is the essential oil stored in the skin of the fruit. Observe how the tangerine smell lingers in the air. Once you've smelled the tangerine, you may feel an intense desire to taste it — deeply, sensuously, and now. But wait. Anticipation is alluring.

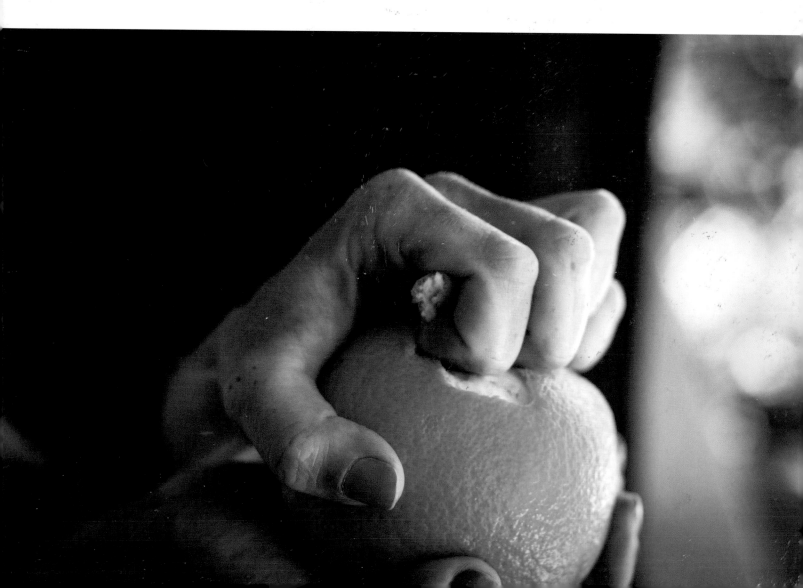

Slowly hold the tangerine with both hands and tear it into two pieces. Note how the fruit is nearly bursting with juices. Touch the flesh of the fruit with your fingers slowly and deliberately, take it in through all of your senses.

Slowly bring one piece up to your lips. Feel the sensation of your lips touching the soft flesh of the fruit. The lips have 100 times more nerve endings than your fingertips. Use them wisely to create a romantic and tasty moment.

Take one bite of the tangerine and let the flavor roll all over the different taste centers on your tongue. Slowly, intentionally, and deliberately suck out the juices. Chew until the tangerine dissolves in your mouth. Slowly swallow. Feel the flavor permeate every part of your body.

Note any sensations in your special tingle zones. Try this exercise with different foods to help you come into awareness.

Here are other foods to try: raspberries, pineapple, papaya, strawberries, blueberries, mango, banana, chocolate, honey, durian, avocado, and passionfruit.

Just think of the fun you and your partner can have rediscovering your senses together. Being mindful of your senses creates electric sensuality that is yours to share.

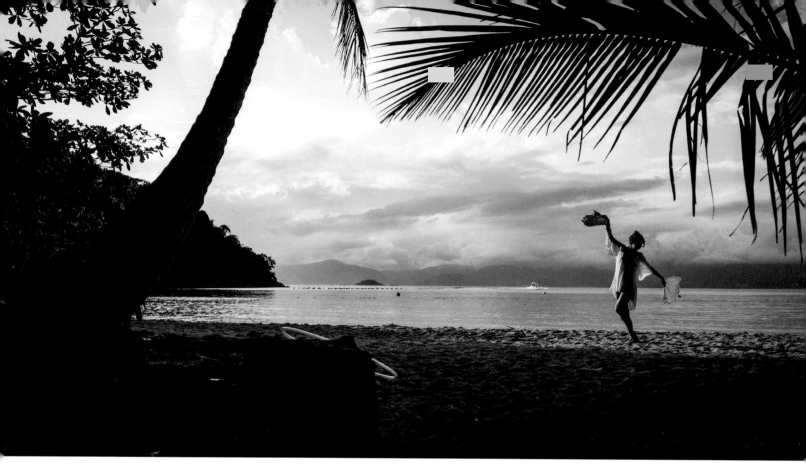

Distill the Essence, Blend the Juice

Distillation *Methods*

In order to distill an essential oil, huge amounts of plant material are needed to extract sometimes minute yields of oils. The cost of the oil depends on the difficulty in obtaining the plant and how much plant material is needed to extract the oil. Some oils cost 10 dollars for five milliliters while others can cost 250 dollars for the same size bottle. As nature would have it, erotics, exotics, and euphorics tend to be more costly. Is pleasure worth the price? This book is about indulging yourself to become a healthier, empowered sensual being. So my answer is a whole-body, hands-in-the-air, emphatic "Yes!" You can easily elicit profound healing and ecstatic responses with essential oils that are incredibly powerful and make for some delicious memories.

Water *Distillation*

In water distillation, plant material is added to a copper still along with water. Heat is added to the still as oil oozes from the plants and rises to the top where it's collected and pure. The water acts as a barrier so the plant material doesn't overheat and destroy the delicate and volatile oils. In steam distillation (the most common form of distillation), plant material is placed in a large still. Water steam is introduced to the plant material in order to separate the aromatic molecules from the plant in vapor form. The steam and aromatic vapor then pass through a cooling rod into tanks where the vapors return to liquid form and create two distinct layers of water and essential oils. At this point, essential oil can be captured and used. In certain distillations, plants like ylang ylang can be distilled up to five times over a 24-hour period.

Hydrosols

Hydrosols or flower waters are a valuable and secondary product produced by the water distillation method. Hydrosols are fascinating because, once consumed, they behave in the body like water. They don't need to be digested like other liquids or foods. They're able to bypass the cell wall and go directly into the nucleus and mitochondria. In doing so, the cell is bathed with the aphrodisiac, immune-boosting, and enlivening qualities of the essential oil at the deepest cellular level. Hydrosols

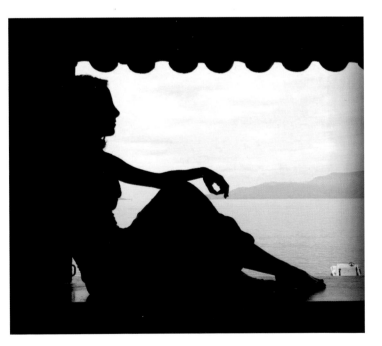

aromatherapy for sensual living   *distill the essence, blend the juice*

are considered to be homeopathic versions of essential oils. They have been used for centuries in cosmetics and food flavoring. Rose water has been a staple of Persian kitchens since the first distillation by Avicenna in the tenth century. By consuming hydrosols (and essential oils) on a regular basis, you can change your molecular structure in order to align with the highest frequencies of plants and flowers.

Absolute *Extraction*

Some plants need special processing in order to extract their oils due to their sensitivity to heat. Absolute extraction uses a solvent (often hexane, a petroleum derivative) or fatty deposit as a base and can pull essential oils that can't be extracted by steam distillation. Jasmine, tuberose, neroli, carnation, labdanum, orange blossom, and rose absolute can be distilled by absolute extraction. Absolutes are perfect for perfume, but shouldn't be used for internal consumption because of the chemicals used.

CO2 *Extraction*

This method of extraction is relatively new. It's similar to absolute extraction, but carbon dioxide is used instead of hexane. The result is an essential oil that has low toxicity and environmental impact and is suitable for consumption. The relatively low temperature of the process and the stability of CO_2 also allow most compounds to be extracted with little damage or denaturing. Vanilla, lavender, sandalwood, cardamom, rose hip, fenugreek, ginger, jasmine, and patchouli can all be extracted by this method.

Expression

Citrus oils such as orange, bergamot, tangerine, grapefruit, lime, and lemon can be extracted by this method. Instead of water or fat, plant material is placed in a device with spikes on the side. The fruits are punctured so that the oil in the skin of the fruit is released. The oil drains down into a machine and is collected and bottled.

Infusion

This is the oldest and simplest form of extracting essential oils and was used throughout ancient Egypt and Rome to obtain the valuable medicinal attributes of the plant. Plant material is submerged in fat or oil for one to four days along with continuous, gentle heat. The medicinal and aromatic qualities of the plant infuse into the oil and are used after straining several times. The disadvantage of this process is that the infusion lacks the concentration of a true essential oil and is susceptible to rancidity.

Essential *Oils Classification*

Essential oils are categorized in many ways. The most common way in aromatherapy and perfume-making is to break down essential oils into top, middle, or base note categories depending on where they appear on the body of the plant, tree, shrub, or root.

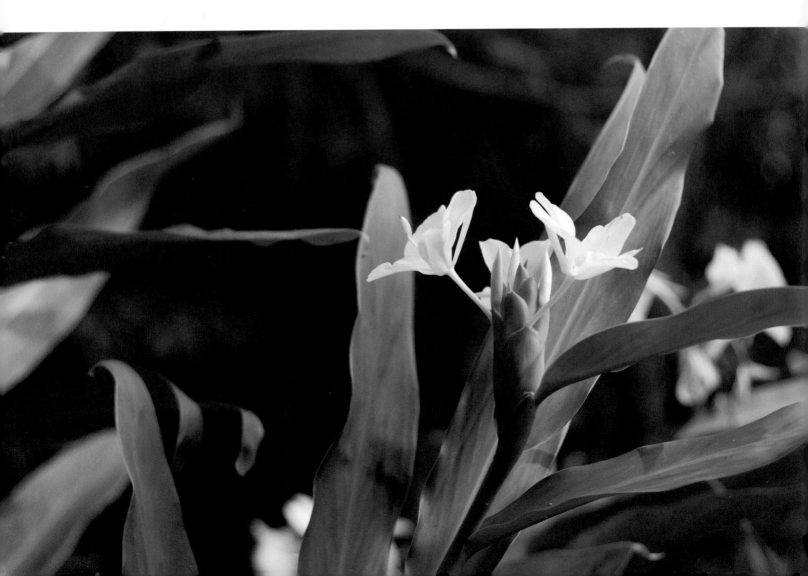

Top notes are generally fruits, twigs, or flowers that appear at the top of a tree. These aromas first hit your nose when smelling a perfume. Most are inexpensive and mood-boosting. They're also the aromas that are the quickest to dissolve and disappear. Top notes are cheerful and have a positive, uplifting energy to them. I use them during the dark days of winter when I need a boost of joy. They're sunshine in a bottle. Some examples are tangerine, lemon, grapefruit, lime, petitgrain, blood orange, and neroli.

Middle notes are usually bushes, grasses, shrubs, barks, flowers, and seeds. They're plants that grow above ground but generally not from the tops of a tree. Most essential oils fall into the middle note category. They linger for longer and provide the body of the blend. Some examples are lavender, black pepper, peppermint, black spruce, cardamom, cypress, caraway, fenugreek, juniper berry, turmeric, eucalyptus, fennel, geranium, thyme, rosemary, manuka, white cedar, marjoram, lemongrass, cinnamon, grand fir, tea tree, and yarrow.

Base notes are obtained from roots, resins, barks, and some flowers. These aromas linger for hours, suspended in time and space. They're deep, heady, and delicious. Base notes are grounding in nature and often help in meditative states. They can easily overpower a blend, so always use with moderation. Base notes tend to be more masculine, too. This is an important aspect if you're blending for a guy and want him to imbibe your aromatic adventure. Sometimes the flowery scents are too overwhelming for his palate and can turn him off. Some base note examples are sandalwood, patchouli, vetiver, ylang ylang, ginger, vanilla, spikenard, and immortelle.

Sometimes oils can fall into more than one category. For instance, marjoram is a classic middle note. It's a shrub that grows close to the ground. However, when you use it in a blend, it can easily take over and behave more like a base note. Some books list basil as a top note, but I use it more as a middle note because it's a small bush and tends to linger longer than other top notes. As you use essential oils, you'll start to see how they behave individually and blended with others to determine their category standing.

There's another category of oils and it's my personal favorite: euphorics. These oils are simply delightful, sensuous, and aromatic. And — surprise, surprise — they induce a state of euphoria and sometimes a narcotic high. Euphorics are total bliss-makers and work powerfully on the endocrine system to release serotonin, dopamine, and other bliss molecules in the brain. The result is that they make you feel soft, warm, inebriated, elevated, excited, swirling, twirling, floating on a cloud, and open to receive deep, delicious desire and attraction. If you ever doubted the power of aromatherapy, spend a couple of hours playing with euphorics. Their force is undeniable. Some examples of euphorics are neroli, vanilla, fenugreek, rose otto, cape chamomile, tarragon, jasmine, tuberose, ylang ylang, sandalwood, ginger, frankincense, and immortelle. They make me swoon with delight.

I recently experimented with neroli on my pulse points. I allowed the oil to penetrate my skin for about twenty minutes before meeting a friend for tea. I felt high in the very best ways. Everything was softer, slower, and more delightful. I found myself in a dreamy state of euphoria for about two hours where I felt I was falling in love, falling through rainbows, and falling into a cloud of feathers and cotton candy. My friend thought it was hilarious to see me so elated in the middle of the day simply by using one drop of an essential oil. It was only then that she began to trust the flowers. She has since become an aroma convert.

Through my twenty-year aroma romance, I've used euphorics in many situations to stimulate, excite, and entice. This is the place where true aromatic sensuality resides. I'm always discovering different ways to adorn myself and/or my lover with euphorics to produce exactly the response I intend. It is an education I am eager to explore.

Extracting *the Essence- Pure Aromatic Artistry*

The process of obtaining essential oils is a beautiful and detailed process involving all aspects of the natural and modern material worlds in graceful union. In order to acquire an essential oil, the plant is adored by the sun and soil for a matter of weeks or years depending on the individual plant material. It's exposed to wind, rain, and sun (and sometimes snow) in the quest to achieve its fullest, most potent beauty. Bees join in to happily carry their pollen to populate other plants and make delicious honey. Flowers burst into existence with an explosion of color, vibrancy, aroma, and beauty.

When they're at their prime and overflowing with nectar, pickers arrive at dusk or dawn to gently and efficiently pick the vast amounts of plant material and swiftly deliver them to the distillation houses. True aromatic artisans distill the flowers (and seeds, needles, roots, barks, leaves, resins, grasses, twigs, and fruit skins) into potent perfumes through time-honored practices and artistic devotion. The perfumes are sold to perfume houses, corporations, and eager aromatherapists, where they're turned into potent and precious combinations, valuable medicines, and sensual delights. The amount of history, energy, intention, integrity, and artistry that is involved humbles me with every drop.

It's always wonderful to receive a dozen roses. Two dozen feels like a luxurious indulgence. Can you imagine six-and-a-half dozen roses all around you?

Did you know it takes eighty rose heads to produce one single drop of rose essential oil? Imagine the heady aroma and vital energy of eighty roses. Envision the colorful vibration and the joy that comes from being surrounded by so much beauty. With essential oils, all of that intention is condensed into one distinct drop of oil. Every single natural element combines in a harmonic dance to provide us with these potent natural medicines. Essential oils are magic sap from the divine.

How *to Blend*

Blending is an art form. It can take years to develop your nose to know which oils blend well together, which ones can take over a blend, or which oils that should never be used for blending. However, it can

be surprisingly easy to make a fully formed blend using some very simple techniques and high quality, medicinal-grade essential oils (from companies like www.purfrequency.com). The best way to get better at anything is through practice and persistence. If your blend smells less than outstanding, allow 24 hours for the oils to mix and mingle and then go back to it. Sometimes it only needs one more drop of a base note, a hint of lavender, or a lift of a top note to make it sing.

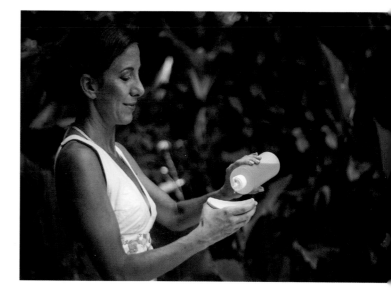

I admit that, through my aromatic love affair, there have been occasions when the mix got too heavy or confusing and I had to give up on the blend. That's okay. It's the path of learning. Very few, if any, people are natural talents on their first try. Give yourself permission to not be perfect on the first round, or ever. Let yourself play. Play is the fountain of youth! Essential oils are patient, loving teachers eager to show you their ways.

There are some basic rules I encourage you to follow when starting on your sensual aromatherapy adventure, even though I am not one to follow the rules. However, start with my recommendations, and once you're comfortable with the basics and safety protocols, and understand how oils blend together and with different carriers, you'll be blending up magic that will make hearts and loins flutter.

Use this blending information in a way that works for you. If you want a deeply grounding blend, use three base notes and one top note for levity. If you're feeling angry and agitated, use mostly top and middle notes with just one drop of a base. If you're feeling out of balance, use mostly middle notes with one top and one base note. The more you use them, the more comfortable you'll be working with them in different strengths and combinations. Trust that aromatherapy is quite safe and there for you to use for health, hot love, and exquisite beauty (with a modicum of knowledge and discretion).

Please follow the rules for internal consumption. Essential oils are very strong and have potent medicinal effects. One to two drops is more than sufficient in a single dose.

As for internal applications, it's absolutely essential to use pure, medicinal, food-grade essential oils from reputable companies that pass the smell test and the United States Food and Drug Administration's GRAS (the acronym for "generally recognized as safe") condition for consumption. Only use steam-distilled or CO_2-extracted oils to ensure that you're taking in valuable medicinals rather than potentially harmful petrochemicals found in absolute extractions. Always check with your health-care provider to ensure that internal applications or the use of essential oils are suitable for your constitution and condition.

For internal applications, I rarely use them neat (undiluted). You can use one drop undiluted and internally, but for many, it's way too intense and can be unpleasant. Neat applications can be used for for bad breath, acute conditions, or a potent immune-boosting blitz (or if you don't have a carrier close

aromatherapy for sensual living *distill the essence, blend the juice*

by). The most pleasurable way of consuming aromatherapy, in my opinion, is diluting one drop in half a teaspoon of raw honey. Other options are ghee, coconut oil, olive oil, sugar cubes, water, coconut water, raw chocolate, on fruit, or in prepared food.

Wait 30 minutes before administering subsequent internal doses, with a maximum of ten drops in a 24-hour period. They're powerful and have the potential to cause harm if too much is taken at one time. There is never an appropriate time to chug a whole bottle.

In so many circumstances, taking essential oils internally is an astounding way to infuse essential oils directly into your cells and drink up divine fluid.

Begin the process of creating your blend with an idea of what you want to make. Do you want your perfume to be effervescent? Deep? Glee-inducing? Do you want a sexy-time blend, a relaxing blend, or an energetic blend? Do you want to soothe your voice, your soul, or your heart? Do you want a medicinal, perfume, or beauty blend? Try to stick to one or two themes because trying to do too much with one blend simply doesn't work and will confuse your nose and body. Once you start smelling and working with the oils, you'll find it's easy to feel out which ones work well together and others that just don't fit. For instance, peppermint and blood orange is an awkward flavor combination. Rose otto and geranium form a loving marriage that sparkles with delight.

I generally make a perfume blend, a loving libation blend, or a room spray in about a 3 percent to 10 percent dilution. In a 5-milliliter bottle (perfume blend), that's between 10 and 20 drops. In a 50-milliliter bottle (room spray), that is about 70 to 100 drops. Just so you know, I like it potent for my pleasures. I tend to use jojoba or spring water for perfume blends. For love butters and massage blends, I use fats such as coconut oil, cacao butter, or shea butter (often combined). For room sprays, I use pure spring water or flower hydrosols as a very luxurious base.

Carrier oils are unscented oils or fats that emolliate an aromatherapy blend and make the essential oil formula last longer. Carrier oils don't evaporate like essential oils and their scent (if any) is less concentrated. Each one has their own unique healing properties that make them wonderful additions to any massage, beauty, or body oiling blend; they give blends gorgeous glide and slide. The same is true for any luscious lover body butter. In moments of exalted bliss, no one wants to be dry like the desert; and there is no need when we have creamy carriers at our bedside. Some of my favorites are:

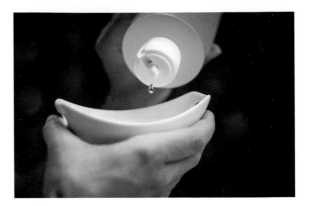

- Jojoba is my go-to carrier oil of choice. It has a long shelf life, and works beautifully with all skin types. I consistently use jojoba in massage and skin-care formulas. This is better for external use.

- Coconut oil smells like tropical heaven. It is a known aphrodisiac that doesn't stain the sheets. It is an edible oil that can be used in any sensual situation. It melts almost instantly and is very beneficial to dry, chapped skin.

- Shea butter is outstanding for wrinkles, excessively dry skin, and stretch marks. It has anti-inflammatory properties along with significant amounts of vitamins A and E (the antioxidant vitamins). The quality and cost of shea butter can drastically vary. Always pay for premium, fresh, pure, and fair-trade shea butter.

- Cacao butter is also known as white chocolate. While I don't recommend eating the butter, I absolutely love it in any skin-care formula. It locks in moisture, smells utterly divine, and is a powerful skin regenerator. Cacao butter can melt in the hands but I prefer to melt it down with other carrier oils. Be sure to buy unrefined, raw, organic cacao butter to receive the positive benefits of the butter.

- Olive oil is a good carrier oil for internal applications, as most people have it available. Olive oil is a monounsaturated fat, meaning it can break down more easily than coconut oil or cacao butter. It is best to store it in the fridge. Olive oil helps prevent cell degeneration in your skin, thus preventing premature aging; however, it will stain sheets and has a pronounced odor, making it too strong for some euphoric or flower oils. It can be useful in hair and mask formulas.

- Ghee is also known as clarified butter. It is a popular fat used in Indian and African cuisine. Ghee, in Ayurveda, is considered one of the most satvic foods, meaning that it promotes positivity, growth, and expansion of consciousness. Ghee can be used internally or placed in the belly button with one drop of essential oil (I love to use jasmine. This is a powerful

aromatherapy for sensual living   *distill the essence, blend the juice*

remedy for many female-related issues). Additionally, it is an excellent massage oil, especially for those with congested bowels or nervous tension.

- Carrot seed oil is an extraordinary oil for skin-care. It is high in antioxidants and very beneficial for puffy, inflamed skin. It contains high levels of beta-carotene and vitamins A, B, C, D, E, and F, and is excellent for mature skin and age spots.

- Hemp seed oil is a powerful polyunsaturated oil. It is very effective for soothing inflammation, boosting neurological and digestive function, and making you feel at ease. Always store hemp seed oil in the fridge as it can break down easily. Additionally, this is best used for internal applications.

- Seabuckthorn is simply divine for skin. It is a reputed anti-inflammatory, incredibly high in vitamin C, and it helps to protect skin against the sun's rays. I have been using seabuckthorn in my skin formulas for over ten years because of its skin regeneration abilities. Always dilute seabuckthorn. Because of its intense orange color, it can stain the skin.

- Rosehip oil is high in vitamin A, a powerful antioxidant. It is known to promote healthy skin cell rejuvenation, helping skin to glow and appear fresh and supple. Rosehip oil works to reduce the appearance of scars, wrinkles, and age spots and is a beneficial immune-supportive oil. It is best just to use a small amount in skin-care formulas.

- Borage oil is an excellent oil to treat damaged, painful, itchy, irritated, inflamed, and acne-prone skin. Much like rosehip oil, it should be used in moderation and with other carriers. It is rather expensive and tends to go rancid quickly. Store it in the fridge and use in moderation.

- Avocado oil is excellent for dry, patchy, inflamed skin. It has a thick, nutty aroma so it is best to dilute it in other carriers. Avocado oil is deeply emollient for the hair. Keep this one in the fridge.

- Pomegranate seed oil is a marvel for skin. It has very high antioxidant values, making it excellent for treating dry, mature, weathered skin. It is one of my favorites for skin-care.

- Baobab oil is grown in Africa and the trees can live up to 1000 years. Baobab is an excellent skin moisturizer and is beneficial for any dry skin formula. It improves elasticity and encourages cell regeneration. Definitely dilute this wonderful oil. A little goes a long way.

aromatherapy for sensual living *distill the essence, blend the juice*

Blending *Basics*

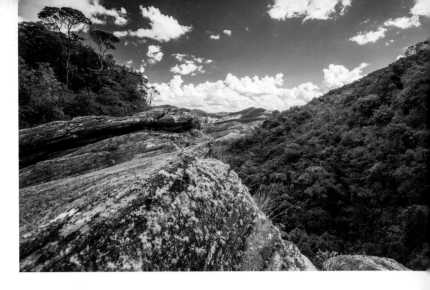

To start your blend, slowly add one drop each of a top, middle, and base note (with the option to delve into the euphorics category). Allow the oils to swirl inside the bottle to develop the full aroma profile, and inhale deeply. You can use perfume tester strips or slivers of watercolor paper to test the aroma after each drop. It will smell differently inside as opposed to outside the bottle when it's exposed to light and air. Smelling between each drop will inform your nose how the oils smell when combined with each other, and you might feel the blend is complete with less. Your nose will tell you when it's done. You'll either feel full and content or like you're aching for just a little bit more. This is also a good reason to put down the bottle, rest, and take time in between drops. Sometimes, in a moment of eager excitement, you'll continue to add drops to the point where the blend just smells rank rather than resplendent.

When it is complete, add water or a carrier oil to finish the blend. If you are making an undiluted blend, be sure to fill the whole bottle with pure essential oils, as your blend will break down much faster if there is a lot of air in the bottle.

Lastly and most importantly, always have a pen and paper handy to write down your blend and the individual drops you used. This is a great learning tool, as you can see where your blend solidified or got off track. It's a real bummer if you forget what you put in your blend when you want to recreate your fabulous perfume in the future.

Slow down, enjoy the process, and allow the blend to evolve without force or speed, and you'll be very happy with the result. Sensuality is about doing things slowly and with the fullest intention of it being your best. Blend on, you sexy siren.

Essential oils are all slightly adaptogenic, meaning that they can bend their shape in order to do what's necessary to suit the situation. If you need levity but only have a base note like sandalwood, it will

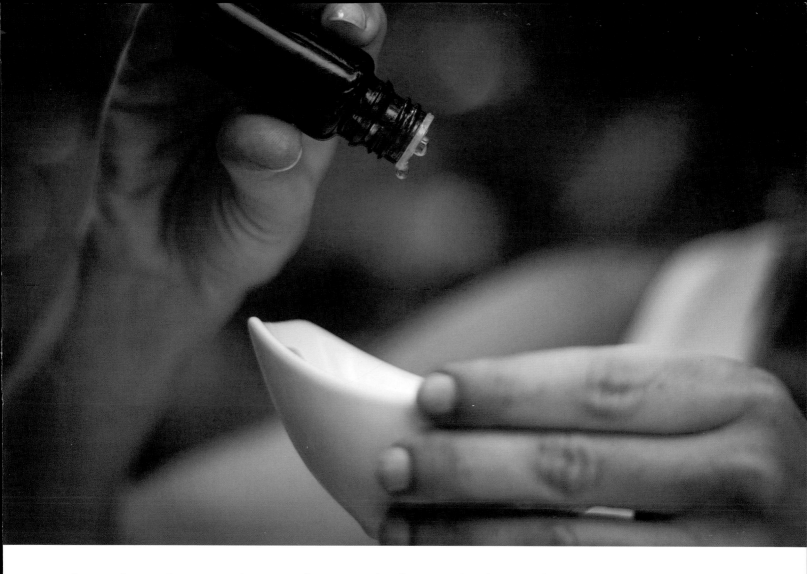

change (sometimes even its aroma) so it can heal you at the deepest level. If you're high-strung and agitated but only have grapefruit, trust that it will cut through the negative emotions and push you into a peaceful place. If you only have cinnamon, laurel, or tuberose, trust that it's the perfect oil for your needs and situation. It's fascinating that plants have an innate understanding of our needs and can alter themselves to help us. I always say that the best oil you have is the one that you have on hand. There's a quiet magic in the plants that is far beyond our realm of understanding. It's one of the reasons that I love essential oils so much.

aromatherapy for sensual living *distill the essence, blend the juice*

Perfect *Pouring*

Pouring oils can be surprisingly tricky. Here are some tips to avoid the dreaded over-pour.

Always hold the pouring bottle at eye level. It may sound overly simple, but it's imperative to the success of your blend. Essential oils are slippery and can come out more quickly or slowly than you expect. Hold the bottle at eye level so you can see every drop. Vetiver empties leisurely. Lavender, on the other hand, decants in a hurry. Bring the pouring bottle and the receiving bottle (or your hand) close to your face to avoid over-pouring or oils splashing out. If your hand is low and you can't see the drops, you can easily tarnish your blend by making it too potent.

Oils like rose absolute, vanilla, or myrrh can pour extremely slowly or even solidify in cooler temperatures. To bring them back to liquid form, put them close to a heater or place them underneath your armpit. Your body temperature is perfect to help them liquefy and roll out. Essential oils break down or evaporate in light, heat, and air, so keep your lids tight and try to keep the bottle away from heat sources (including close to a hot shower). If the oil still doesn't want to move after a few minutes, pop off the top with a pair of scissors and insert a toothpick to gather the oil. It will thin out once it's in carrier oil.

Blending *styles*

When I teach aromatherapy and blending, I talk to people about different ways to produce a complete, rounded, fully formed aroma creation. I ask people to share their learning styles and if they see themselves as visual, auditory, emotional, numerical, or physical learners. What are you? By knowing what type of learner you are, you can create a blend that best suits your natural skills.

Aromatherapy, especially sensual aromatherapy, is easily guided through our connection to our senses. I'm primarily a visual learner. When I blend, I often see a section of the color spectrum, a shape (often an oval, sphere, or a hexagon), or a landscape like a forest, a wildflower field, or the ocean. Sometimes I hear a musical chord or feel an emotion I want to create. When I blend, I "paint" with the oils to fill in the shape, sound, or landscape I see in my mind. It's a form of synesthesia, or a mixing of the senses.

If you are open, you'll learn to see, hear, feel, and understand the oils as you learn their individual personalities. It's the same as meeting a person with whom you instantly click and then spend quality time developing a deep and meaningful relationship. It's not difficult, as the oils are eager to show off their stuff (they are such flirts). They just need time and attention. I invite my students to think about what they want in their blend so they can "paint" the smell, "hear" the complete aroma chord, or "emote" their way through the process. I find that when I stop thinking and go with feeling, I always produce a better, more dynamic and complete blend.

Sometimes the oils will alter their shape, color, sound, or appearance when combined with other oils. Lavender with rose is a shimmery, luminescent love bomb. But when blended with peppermint, lavender is a workhorse that's committed to curing shock and trauma.

Another way to blend is based on the number of oils in the concoction and knowing what they'll bring to the blend. I learned this method from an extremely talented herbalist friend, Roger Lewis, and have been very pleased with the results. Here's an overview:

- **One** oil helps connect us to source energy. It's powerful to connect to one oil. Ask a question, wait patiently, and receive a response. The oils have infinite intelligence to help you.

- **Two** oils will help solidify a connection to another person. It also imparts balance and yin/yang energy. There's a Chinese expression that says: "Good things come in pairs." Blending with two oils will ensure good things.

- **Three** oils help deepen a mind, body, and spirit connection, or impart information regarding a past, present, or future situation. Blending with three oils also allows you to use a base, middle, and top note to create balance in the blend.

- **Four** oils help form solidity like the four legs of a chair. Blending with four oils helps to convey order, organization, and where ideas are manifested into reality. If you're looking to execute a plan or idea, blending with four oils will help to solidify it.

- **Five** oils help heal family relations and impart the five elements (metal, water, fire, wind, earth), giving the blend wholeness and stability. Using five oils also relates to

aromatherapy for sensual living *distill the essence, blend the juice*

freedom in action and potent creativity. It will help to ensure that your blend will be one of progression and passion. I often use five oils in my blends.

- **Six** oils help to bring in protection and self-healing. This helps to gain clarity on difficult decisions. It symbolizes responsibility and service, which need to be achieved through love and nurturing. Six is innately feminine, watery, and yin-like.

- **Seven** oils help cure imbalances in the chakra system and support spiritual awakening and development. Seven is generally considered lucky and a powerful number to use in your blend. It's also one of my favorites.

- **Eight** oils speak to the infinity of the universe, personal power, and inner strength. Using eight oils brings in the great karmic equalizer. I often use eight oils to charge the blend with sovereignty and abundance.

- **Nine** oils help with independence, resilience, and deep inner courage. Nine oils bring in consciousness, skill, and tolerance. This number involves universal love and is probably the most romantic of all the numbers.

A blend with more than seven oils is difficult. I often stop around four or five. Experiment with different numbers to see what works well for you. At the beginning, less is more. When you're first learning to blend, I recommend working with a maximum of three oils so you can learn how they work in combination with each other and receive the magnitude of information in just a couple of aromas. Nature is vast.

The most common mistake that I see in my classes is that students use too many oils in a blend. It's natural to want to feast on all of the glorious options that are available but, sweet sensual lover, less is more.

For one of my first blends, I wanted to make the most sensual, erotic, and potent blend imaginable. I gleefully added drops of jasmine, ylang ylang, rose otto, neroli, and vanilla, thinking that if I combined all the erotic oils I would be an unstoppable man-slayer. The idea was good but the result was horrible. It smelled heavy and overdone. It stunk and ultimately sank. When you first start learning how to play with oils, limit yourself to three or four choices. Specifically in sensual aromatherapy, I use two or three oils as a maximum.

Without a great degree of experience with natural perfumes, too many scents can confuse and even aggravate your lover. Aggravation isn't what I imagine you're looking for. Simplicity, in a blend as in life, is the key.

Massage *Blend*

If you're making a massage blend, start with one tablespoon of carrier oil and then add one drop from the top, middle, and base categories. Balance is the key to an effective and memorable massage. If you're trying to evoke a sexy response, experiment with an additional drop from the euphorics category. Continue to add one drop from each category to strengthen the blend. Remember that middle notes tend to be the body of the blend, with top notes and base notes used for accents and gravity. It's quite important to smell the blend in between each drop. Essential oils are amazingly powerful. One extra drop can change an entire blend and make it too heavy or full. Massage blends are between a 3 percent and 15 percent dilution with a carrier oil.

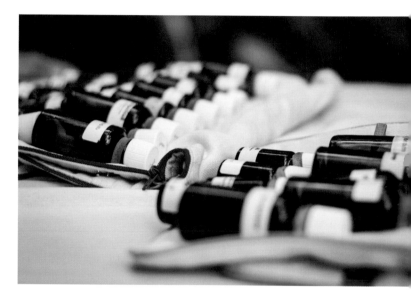

Room *Sprays*

Room sprays are an easy and inexpensive way to experiment with essential oils and a healthy alternative to chemical-laden and toxic room sprays and wall plug-ins. Depending on the size of the bottle, use between 30 and 75 drops along with spring water — between 10 percent and 20 percent dilution. I use smaller bottles so I can change the aroma in my home regularly. I tend to stick to mostly middle notes for room sprays. It makes the indoor environment tranquil.

Culinary oils, especially from the citrus family, are particularly good for room sprays. In my twenty years of working and healing with aromatherapy, I've yet to meet anyone who dislikes tangerine, grapefruit, or lemon. However, if you're scenting your space for an aromatic lover, I suggest using deeper and headier notes like ylang ylang, vetiver, sandalwood, and/or some of the euphorics. It will instantly calm any pre-date nerves and help you and your lover be open and receptive to meet each other in love.

I especially love fenugreek in room sprays. It has a pleasant, sweet, and welcoming aroma that's perfect for setting the mood.

Using essential oil room sprays will also help to purify and detoxify the air in your home.

Cologne

In my opinion, commercial cologne is some of the most putrid and offensive-smelling garbage on the planet. There's nothing that turns me off faster than getting close to a man only to retreat because he smells of a synthetic, caustic aroma bomb. I set out to change this in my own small way. In my mid-twenties, I created a blend that was my dream man in a bottle. It included 20 percent vanilla, 15 percent vetiver, 15 percent bergamot, 10 percent petitgrain, 20 percent sandalwood, 10 percent tangerine and 10 percent patchouli. "Mojo for Men" has long been a huge hit with all my male clients. It was once described as "lady bait." That still makes me smile.

Deodorant

Conventional deodorants are full of sulfates, aluminums, and toxins that are very harmful to the delicate underarm skin. These chemicals leach directly into the lymph system, increasing the toxic load in the whole body. Luckily, nature has the answer to stifle the stench and help us smell glorious.

To make your own deodorant, start with sandalwood as the carrier oil and base. Sandalwood has an amazing affinity with the armpits and helps both men and women smell radiant. There's almost nothing I love more than the smell of a man, clean from the shower, emitting his natural, manly aroma. However, when some men start doing their manly things, they can smell slightly less fragrant. Sandalwood blends with both men and women's unique aroma to produce something sensual, aromatic, deep, and delicious. Sandalwood also contains a phyto-androgen that blends beautifully with our natural aroma and helps to disinfect unpleasant and unkind aromas.

Add 5 percent to 10 percent of a blend into the sandalwood oil carrier. Oils that blend beautifully with sandalwood are rose otto, lavender, palo santo, vetiver, ylang ylang, geranium, patchouli, fenugreek, and neroli. Be creative. Try to stay away from oils that may cause a reaction to sensitive skin, including vanilla, black pepper, clove, ginger, cinnamon, and citrus oils. Trust that our bodies are supposed to sweat. Antiperspirant goes against our natural detoxification pathways and can clog delicate lymph tissue. Sweating is that much more beautiful when it's graced by the healing power of flowers. I imagine (and hope) that you'll never go back to those toxic white sticks again.

Keep *it Clean*

We live in a chemical-saturated world. There are 70,000 synthetic chemicals that we're in contact with virtually all the time. Our bodies simply aren't designed to understand or process elements that are outside of nature. The result is our detoxification pathways get clogged up by fake stuff, making it more difficult to sniff out the good stuff (and the reason why you may sneeze when initially smelling authentic essential oils). Our internal environments can often be more toxic than outdoors. In using chemicals, especially in the home, we're adding to our overall toxic load. A burdened toxic load will give way to chronic disease, inflammation of organs and tissues, and preventable illness in the body. We can do a lot to correct the balance by sticking with what's real, authentic, and truly beautiful.

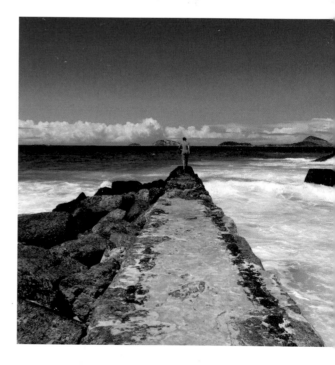

One of the most important ways to transform our living environments is to clean without chemicals. It's easy; just ask your grandmother. To clean my floors, I use hot water, Dr. Bronner's castile liquid soap, and white cedar or black spruce essential oil. I use natural dish and laundry soap and add rosemary,

Douglas fir, and/or lavender to improve cleaning ability and enhance smell. I clean my bathroom with tea tree, lemon, baking soda, and natural abrasive soap when necessary.

You can additionally improve your capacity to smell and accelerate your health with a few lifestyle alterations. First and foremost, be a scent sleuth. Chemical fragrance hides in many, often unexpected, things. Go through your bathroom, make-up bag, kitchen, and laundry room to remove all synthetic fragrances from your home.

Consider a lifestyle makeover. Choose natural over synthetic, lose weight, feel better, and have more energy for love and life. Avoid phlegm-forming foods like pasteurized dairy products (especially ice cream), fried foods, excessive meat consumption, caffeine products, sugar, and wheat. Drink more spring water to remove toxins from the body. You can improve your ability to smell by eating organic food. Pesticides, herbicides, and fungicides all also contribute to your toxic load and cause inflammation in the body. The result is the delicate tissues in your nostrils will also be swollen (limiting your capacity to smell).

For an easy custom soap recipe, start with a natural, gentle, scent-free liquid soap. Pour out ⅛ of an inch of soap. With any aroma addition, be sure to shake (not stir) the bottle to incorporate the blend into the liquid soap.

- For a fresh and clean scent, fill it up with an essential oil blend of 25 percent black spruce, 25 percent rosemary, 25 percent lemon, 20 percent lavender, and 5 percent patchouli.

- For a soft, feminine essential oil blend, add 25 percent lavender, 20 percent cape chamomile, 10 percent vanilla, 15 percent geranium, 15 percent sandalwood, and 15 percent cardamom.

- For a macho-man aroma, combine 20 percent sandalwood, 15 percent patchouli, 20 percent vetiver, 20 percent white cedar, 15 percent Douglas fir, and 10 percent grapefruit.

I'm always tickled by my ability to pick up aromas in a room long before anyone else. I have a special "smell-o-vision" enhanced by my years of healthy living and essential oil usage. This skill has come in handy to detect the alluring scent of love, pick up delicate flavors in food, or discern different essential oils in a blend.

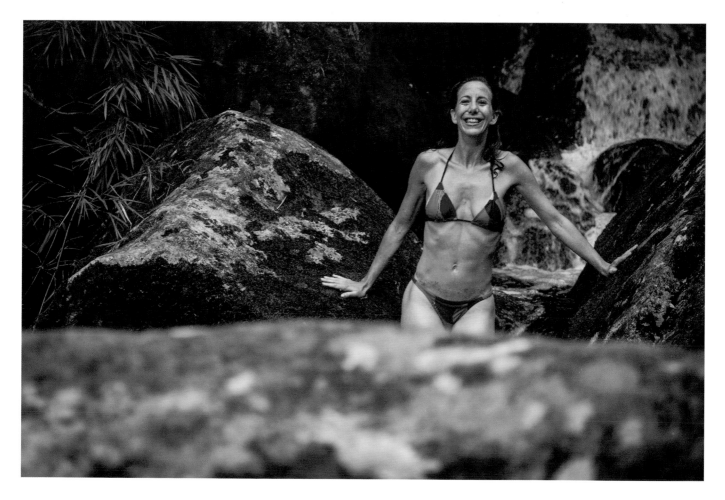

Other *Tempting and Effective Practices*

There are constantly new and innovative ways to include essential oils in my aromatic life. Here are some other methods to try:

- Inhalation: Drop one or two undiluted drops of oil onto your hands and cover your mouth and nose. Inhale deeply (with eyes closed) for several minutes to allow the oils to penetrate your lungs, brain, and blood system. This is one of the easiest and most direct methods of application.

- Neat application: Drop one or two drops of oil on skin for such specific purposes as disinfecting the skin, anointing skin with pure perfume, or treating a pimple or cold sore.

- Compress: Add 10 drops of pure essential oil to a bowl of warm or cool water. Soak a cloth with the mixture and wring it out. Apply it to the head, kidneys, stomach, or sore and tender muscles. Compresses tame mild fevers, indigestion, muscle strain or pain, inflammation, and edema, and also help intensify contractions in labor. Replace the cloth every few minutes for at least an hour.

- Salve: Add three or four drops of essential oil to a natural salve blend and mix well. Apply to areas such as the lungs to treat congestion and chest colds, or behind the ears and down the neck to calm earaches. I like to add a covered hot water bottle on top of the salve to deepen the healing.

- Suppository: Add three to five drops of essential oils to one tablespoon of coconut oil. Slowly melt together over a double boiler and mix well. Cool slightly and add the combination to vegetarian capsules or pour it into mini ice cube trays and place in the fridge for four hours to allow the suppository to form. Apply suppositories as needed to treat specific conditions.

- Vaporizer Pen: Add one to three drops of essential oils into pure, non-palm, food-grade vegetable glycerin (corn vegetable glycerin is preferred). Pour the combination into a 1- to 1.5-milliliter vaporizer pen. Inhale five to ten breaths slowly in order to receive the effect of the oils into your circulatory system. Repeat as necessary throughout the day, with a maximum of six servings a day.

- Humidifier: Add twenty drops of essential oils to a large pot of water. Simmer on low until the water has evaporated. This is an excellent method to remove pathogens from the air or scent the home with powerful aromatherapy. Alternatively, add twenty drops to a plug-in humidifier. Use this method every other day.

- Radiators: Add ten drops of essential oils to water in a large bowl. Submerge towels in the water. Wring them out and place them on hot radiators to moisten dry air with aromatic delights.

- In socks: Add one or two drops of warming essential oils to half a tablespoon of coconut oil. Mix well and apply to feet. Wait five minutes and cover with woolly socks. This method will effectively warm the body on the coldest winter day. You will have happy, softened and improved circulation.

- In laundry soap: Add 50-100 drops of a clear-colored disinfecting or euphoric aromatherapy blend to a large bottle of liquid laundry soap. Shake well and use normally in the washing machine. This method isn't intended for delicate fabrics.

- Dryer sheet: Add ten drops of essential oils to a damp cloth and toss it in the dryer along with wet clothes. Use the dryer normally. It's a beautiful way to impart essential oils into fabrics for long-lasting, non-toxic aroma.

- Mop floors: Add ten drops of tree, citrus, or herbaceous oils to hot water and soap. Mop normally.

- Bathroom cleaning: Add five drops to toilet bowl/bath/sink and scrub down any accumulated dirt. This is a popular and easy method if there's an unpleasant bathroom odor.

- Tea: Add one drop of food-grade, steam-distilled essential oil to a teaspoon of honey. Mix well and then add the combination to a cup of hot water. Stir. Drink as you would a normal tea.

- Tissue: Add one to three drops of essential oils to a tissue and place it in your bra or shirt pocket. Inhale aromatic beauty throughout the day to increase the peace. You can also place the tissue on a pillow before you go to sleep to help ease anxiety, improve sleep, and ensure peaceful dreams. Lavender, cape chamomile, and/or marjoram are effective for sleep.

- Lozenges: In a bowl mix two tablespoons of creamed raw honey, ten drops of cardamom essential oil, and enough slippery elm powder to form a thick mixture. Form the mixture in a long tube. Cut into small pieces. Place in the freezer overnight. Store in the fridge.

- Writing paper: Add a few drops of essential oils to your hand and rub them over pretty paper. Allow it to dry and send your lover an aromatic message. Alternatively, saturate a small strip of watercolor paper with essential oils and place it in the envelope. It is quite delightful to open up a letter and receive an aromatic surprise.

Symptom *to Cure*

All essential oils carry potent medicinal properties. I've used them to stop a herpes outbreak, tame violent menstrual cramps, reduce a fever, heal severe burns, stop a serious asthma attack, and of course, thrill a lover with absolute delight. Their uses and beauty are infinite.

When I was teaching aromatherapy in Japan, I was struck down with a very fast and intense head cold. I was quite ill and had to figure out the best course of action so I could teach a few hours later. I used six drops of an immune blend on raw chocolate internally over twenty minutes and I was very close to perfect when it came time to teach.

On another occasion, I was in the Brazilian jungle. A friend stepped on a red ant hill and was immediately swarmed and stung. Big, red, painful welts appeared all over her feet and lower legs within seconds. I administered peppermint to calm the redness and cool the pain, followed by lavender to treat the skin, and then frankincense to soothe the skin. The result was a profound recovery nearly 24 hours later.

In yogic tradition, the sense of smell is connected to the root chakra. This chakra, found at the base of the spine, helps us feel grounded and connected to our surroundings. It governs security, passion, trust, and relationships with money, home, and career. When the root chakra is balanced, we feel safe, connected to the earth, and in touch with our bodies. When it's not we are anxious, easily stressed, or constantly worried. Nature has the solution! Inhale rich, heady aromas, such as sandalwood or patchouli (base notes). They will tone and support this chakra. By focusing on our sense of smell and breathing deeply, we can help to calm frazzled nerves and be more at peace and grounded. Isn't it amazing that we can smell our way to more peace and spiritual development?

Deepening *Sensuality: Full Body Cardamom Saturation*

One of the best ways to get acquainted with essential oils is to do a full body immersion. I describe it as a live embalming where you use every method imaginable to fully saturate yourself with oils and truly understand their power and potency. With cardamom (or any edible erotic oil), use as many oil and/or herb variations as possible over a 24-hour period to get the full toe-curling effect. Use your creativity. Notice your special tingle zones and where the oils flow in your body. I've used this methodology in my personal practice and noticed that there's an undeniable force that is created for all those who smell me after an immersion. It's a rare and special magic, and one that's utterly fun to use.

Some examples of immersion are:

- Add drops to your mop water

- Drink tea with the herb

- Do a hair rinse with the herb tea

- Steam inhalation

- Clay mask with added oils

- Mist your room, sheets, and skin with essential oils and water

- Massage blended oil into hands, feet and hair

- Add a drop to your smoothie

- Use body oils

- Take a bath with cardamom and coconut oil

- Wash your sheets and clothes with the oil and laundry soap (use a clear oil)

- Anoint all your pulse points with pure oil and tap the points to get the essential oils coursing through your bloodstream

aromatherapy for sensual living *distill the essence, blend the juice*

- Anoint your lady petals with the essential oil and jojoba. (Avoid using black pepper, cinnamon, cassia bark, or peppermint on your petals. These will cause burning, itching and even chafing on the most sensitive of skins.)

- Feed your lover high quality (preferably raw) chocolate with one drop of essential oil. Do it slowly, intentionally, and in small pieces so that it's eaten out of the palm of your hand. The combination of chocolate with oils is a pure bliss-maker.

aromatherapy for sensual living   *distill the essence, blend the juice*

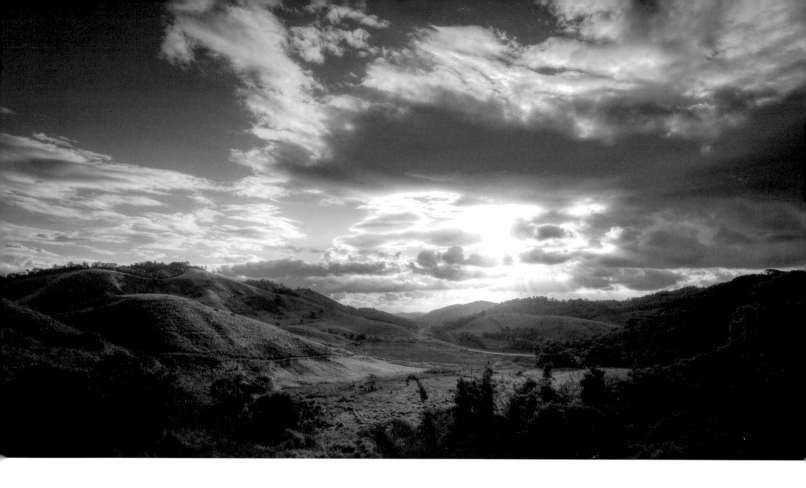

Fabulous Pheromones: The Smell of Sex

"When we smell another's body, it is that body that we are breathing in through our mouth and nose, that we possess instantly, as it were in its most secret substance, its own nature. Once inhaled, the smell is the fusion of the other's body and my own."

– Jean-Paul Sartre

In an effort to make my purpose for being in Brazil understood to those who didn't speak English, I said in simple Portuguese: "Estou escrevendo um livro sobre o aroma e sexo." That means "I'm writing a book on smell and sex." Without fail, there was an excited giggle and understanding that smell and sex have an intimate and palpable relationship.

We're creatures driven by smells. It's something we intimately understand. More than visual, our system of navigation is smell-oriented. Pheromones are emitted to sniff out a potential mate. It's primeval, so why fight something that's innate? We can smell someone's health, vitality, and compatibility through a complex and mysterious alchemical process, and most of it's so subtle that it happens without our knowledge. Pheromones serve a primitive biological purpose grounded in evolutionary mate selection, and they affect behavior in humans and animals on a subconscious level.

Pheromones were first defined in 1959. The word "pheromone" is derived from the Greek words "pherein" (to bear or transport) and "hormone" (to stimulate or excite). They contribute to who we find attractive, but also have other purposes in the animal kingdom, including signaling and warning, forming social groups, and coupling behaviors. Their purpose is to boost attraction and convey information. Above all, pheromones allow for a form of silent and purely chemical communication between two living beings. It's sexy power in action.

While "your pheromones drive me wild" may not be a common pick-up line, it explains the hot magnetism that pulls two people together and ultimately leads to love, bonding, and steamy and erotic moments. Love at first sniff? Do the smell test. The better the person smells, the better he/she is for you. The nose is wise. Trust it.

One of the benefits of kissing is that we get close enough to detect pheromones. Skin to skin contact also releases pheromones that trigger desire. Perhaps that's the innate problem with online dating; you need to smell potential love-friends to feel out their compatibility. In humans, pheromones originate in special glands near the armpits, where they're released as sweat; or near the genital region. There are subtle smells emitted from pubic hair, so perhaps going for a full Brazilian bikini wax isn't the best way to attract the love you crave.

Pheromones *in the Floral and Animal World*

"Do you want me to tell you a secret? The flowers attract the most beautiful lover with their sweet smile and scent." – Rumi

Plants release and exude pheromones as their form of communication — a dance between giver and receiver. Flowers emit potent perfume in an effort to bewitch bees into carrying their pollen. The bee graciously accepts the floral nectar offering. Drunk on flower dust, they fly off and spread the flower syrup far and wide, making honey moonshine for us to enjoy. The flowers and bees work together synergistically and the result is a beneficial and scintillating relationship.

The bee produces honey and the flower receives the necessary boost to blossom. It's balance, teamwork, and partnership at its finest. The reason why flowers smell so enchanting is credited to their emitting plant pheromones to attract love-making bees. Bees also pass pheromones on to the flower to indicate they've already visited and the flower is out of nectar. Insects also play a role in this sacred

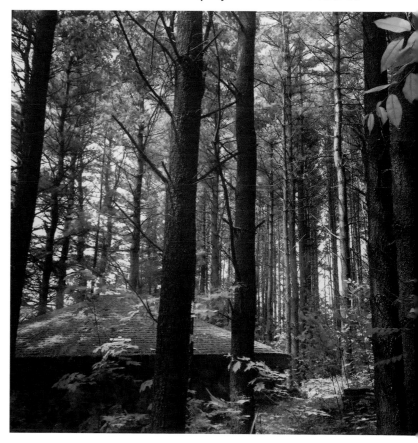

aphrodisiac of nature by releasing a pheromone into the air to signal their readiness to copulate. Oh the magic.

Your pheromones are unique to you and serve as an attractant signature that conveys pertinent information to potential mates. They can't be bottled or duplicated. This isn't to say that the perfume industry hasn't tried with bottled synthetic pheromone spray. Additionally, unnatural body washes, antibacterial soaps, and stinky antiperspirants aren't ideal either, as they prevent the release of sweat and inhibit the natural flow of pheromones. Your armpits are broadcasting important and juicy information. Don't let that go to waste. Go with a natural aromatic deodorant as an alternative.

If perfume's desire is to enhance our scent, only to make us smell false, I invite you to consider using authentic essential oil botanicals that contain compelling and inviting flower pheromones. You can better your unique personal aroma by choosing natural products over heavily (and synthetically) perfumed bath and body products. No matter how good you look, no one will want to be with you if you smell bad. Going au naturel is an opportunity to blend our personal fragrance and that of flirting flowers to help us smell like the sweetest peach.

Deepening *your personal aroma*

Each one of us has a unique personal aroma. It's a powerful clue as to one's biology, health, food choices, exercise, and hygiene. When we practice a healthy lifestyle and make positive choices, we naturally smell and feel better. Some say vegans taste better and smokers taste like ashtrays. I believe you smell and taste better when you take care of yourself and actively promote your health with good daily habits. Sensuality is all about feeling, looking, and emanating your best.

I once briefly dated a man who was perfect on paper, but I just couldn't get over that he smelled of musty old clothes and odiferous blue cheese. For my distinct biology, it was a devastating aroma

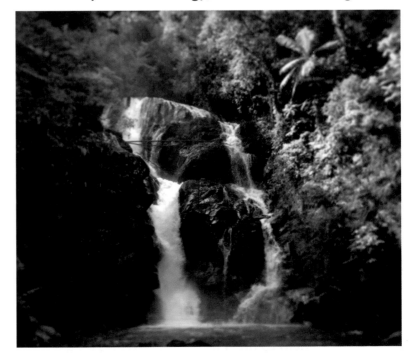

bomb. Needless to say, it didn't last long. Another time, I fell in love with a man by simply smelling his hair before I even got to know him. There was just a certain something about his scent that totally lured me in. Additionally, I've smelled the scarf of the man I loved and it instantly ignited my special tingle zones. Our nose always knows who is a good biological match, unless of course you are on the birth control pill. The pill blocks a woman's ability to decipher pheromones and suitable compatibility. This is one more reason to get off the pill.

I encourage people in my workshops to learn about the aromas of others by being blindfolded and smelling the wrists, necks, and even armpits of the other participants. It's a highly intimate activity that certainly breaks the ice. This activity develops our smell vocabulary and acuity. After the exercise, I invite people to describe what they smelled and list their desire accordingly. It's a fascinating experiment that has even led to a date or two.

The key to distillation is that if you don't like their smell, it isn't going to be a great pairing.

Deepening *Sensuality: How to Heal a Broken Heart*

Heartbreak . . . we've all been there and, ubiquitously, it sucks. The physical pain the body feels when we're separated from our lover is visceral and real. Sometimes it can feel like our broken heart is never going to mend. It's such a tender and intelligent organ and, luckily and thankfully, capable of repair.

I've used this protocol in clinic and personally for years. It's incredibly powerful and deeply nurturing. Trust that the flowers can help ease the pain and provide you with vital support at a time when you are most vulnerable and raw. Use this protocol as often as needed for a long as you need. I assure you that you will feel a shift.

- Eat one drop of steam-distilled rose otto essential oil on half a teaspoon of raw honey two to three times a day. Direct the energy of the oil to your heart to heal any broken, bruised, or battered parts of you.

- In your mind's eye, create an infinity symbol starting at your heart. Direct the symbol into the center of the earth, loop it up through your heart, and then up through the center of the sun. Cycle the energy back through your heart and back again into the earth. Continue the infinity current under you until you feel grounded.

- Drink organic rose petal and hawthorn tea throughout the course of the day.

- Bathe in rose otto or rose absolute and sea salt three times a week. The sea salt will help to draw out the stress and impurities associated with negative emotions.

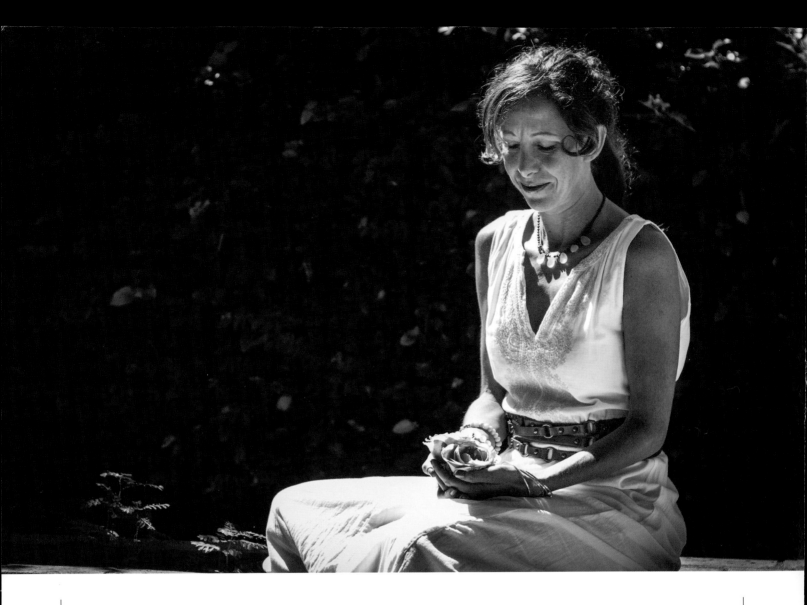

- Wear rose quartz crystals in your bra, on a necklace, or as close to your heart as possible. You can also add them to your bath or drinking water.

- Wear pink and/or green clothing, especially on the upper torso or around the heart. These colors help tone the heart in the chakra system. By harnessing the power of color, you're treating the damaged organ and helping it to repair.

- Lie down on the ground with your heart touching the earth (it's best to do this on the grass) and allow all the sad, hurt, angry, and rejected feelings to bleed out of your body. Mama nature is there to receive you unconditionally. This feels amazing.

- Trick your body into being happy by using positive affirmations. Use potent and positive visualizations of you returning to your buoyant and blissful self or finding a love that's right for you.

- Use the rose meditation twice a day. (See page **92** for more on this.)

- Finally, know that time heals all wounds. You're the living embodiment of the divine light and your birthright is to shine. Trust that the wisdom of the universe is leading you to the right love with the right person who will cherish you and not break your heart.

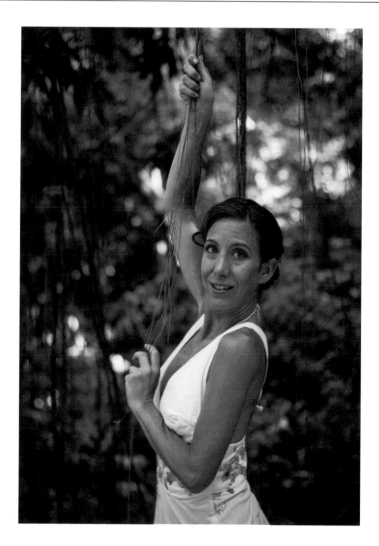

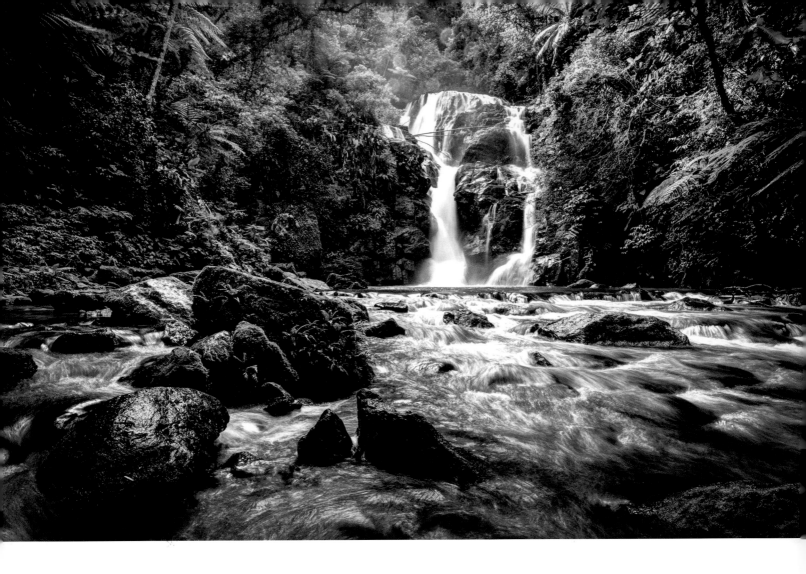

Bewitching Beauty Rituals

"Odors have a power of persuasion stronger than that of words, appearances, emotions, or will. The persuasive power of an odor cannot be fended off, it enters into us like breath into our lungs, it fills us up, imbues us totally. There is no remedy for it." – Patrick Suskind, *Perfume: The Story of a Murderer*

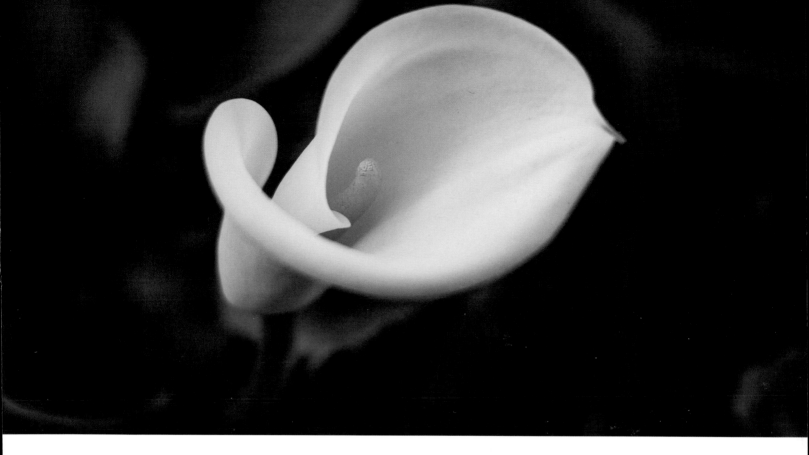

In our busy and demanding lives, our self-care and radiant beauty can fall to the bottom of our priority list. Relinquish the glorification of busy and the impossibly high standards women are forced to meet. These arbitrary standards don't create the balance we need to be the flower. Let's try something new.

Beauty is a woman who holds her own.

In order to take care of the myriad of responsibilities we women have, we, first and foremost, must take care of ourselves. Your beauty is like a muscle in need of strength. What better way to honor the divine in you than to spend time adoring and adorning your body temple? Brush your hair lovingly with oils for five minutes. Commit to a daily bathing practice with essential oils and candles. Practice taking full, deep, cleansing, aromatic breaths into all parts of your body. Your self-love sets an example for others to enjoy this moment, sip in beauty, and simmer down. Beauty is a slow, sensual burn.

Self-care isn't a needless indulgence but mandatory in order to live a healthy, vibrant, productive life that honors the divine feminine. Nature provides us with countless tools to enhance our beauty. As we let the artificial, synthetic, adulterated, and chemical clutter fall away, we are left with authentic botanicals that genuinely boost our beauty and celebrate natural radiance.

Many of us have experimented with a homemade clay mask, exfoliated with sugar, or added lemon to our hair to create natural highlights. We keep going back to time-tested potions and concoctions because they work and are safe. The great news is that essential oils can take those practices deeper and make them even more potent, healing, and nurturing. Nature is on our side to make us our most juicy. Bless the mama.

This section is designed to help you, on every level of your being, *be the flower.*

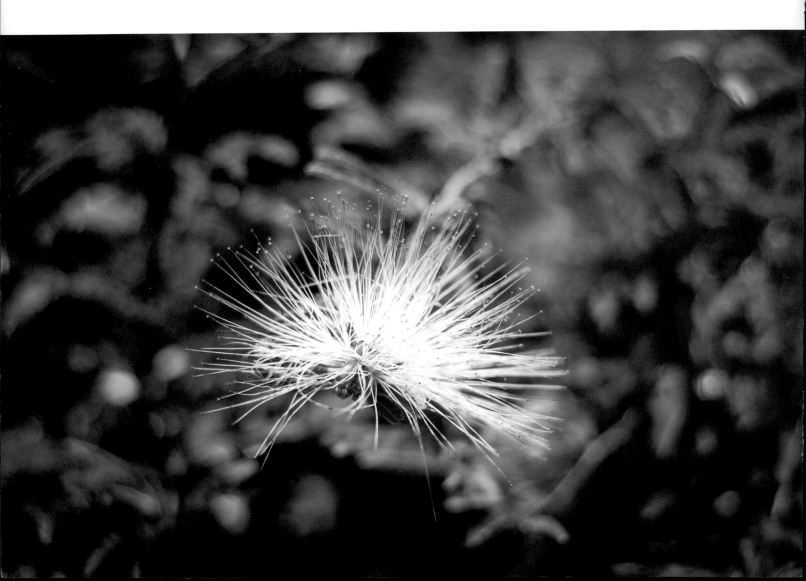

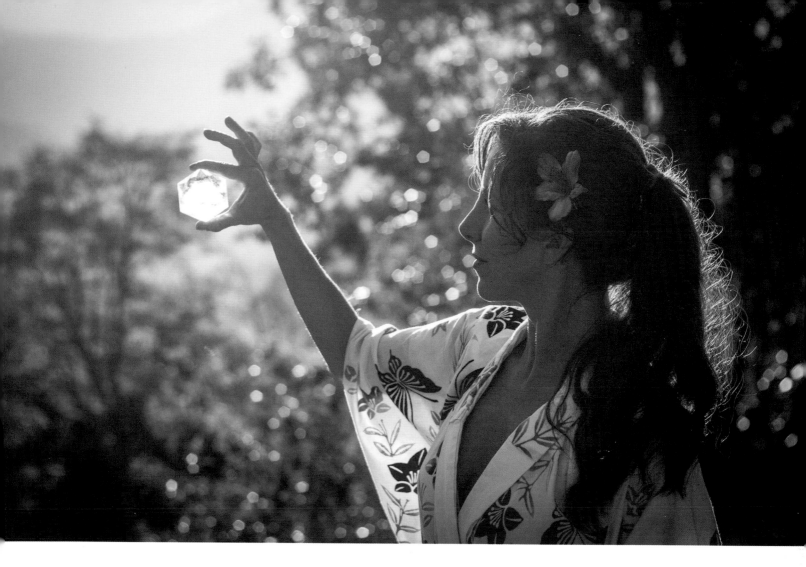

Body *Oiling*

Body oiling is an ancient technique used in Ayurvedic medicine — the oldest system of medicine on the planet. Our skin is aching to be cared for, yearning to be touched, and begging for natural medicines as opposed to the failed promises of synthetically perfumed potions and commercial creams. Nature always knows best.

According to Ayurvedic medicine, body oiling boosts the immune system, relaxes the mind and central nervous system, and makes muscles and tissues supple. Not surprisingly, body oiling feels really good on the skin, especially received from a dreamy hunky lover. Pure essential oils combined with luxurious carrier oils deeply nourish skin and actively reduce wrinkles, bruises, burns, blemishes, age spots, and skin discolorations.

Body oiling is a totally luxurious process that yields tremendous results both for your skin and your entire being. I like to body oil when I first get out of the shower and my skin is still warm and wet. Start by choosing your favorite carrier oil such as jojoba, cacao butter, rose hip oil, baobab oil, coco babacu, coco cream, and/or shea butter combined with an essential oil blend of your choice. Aim for a blend of ten drops in two tablespoons of carrier oil.

Some effective essential oils to add to your body oil blend are:

- Juniper berry, basil, lavender – improves circulation and detoxification pathways

- Ylang ylang, bergamot, cinnamon – heightens sexual desire and energy

- Cardamom, vanilla, immortelle – a stimulating euphoric blend

- Jasmine, hay, blood orange, black pepper – excellent blend for both men and women

- Lemongrass, lemon, lavender, rosemary – cleansing, energizing, purifying

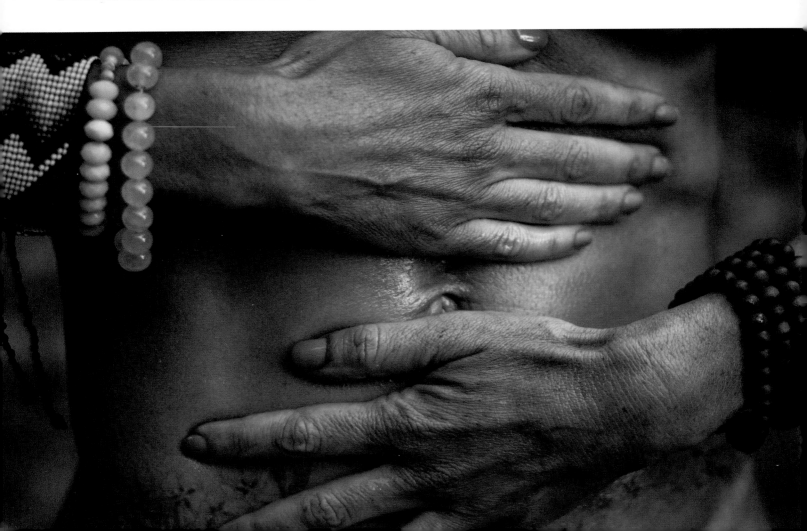

Grace your body with a massage of long, firm, and loving strokes up the legs, over the stomach and buttocks, around the back and over the breasts, completing with arms — always moving in the direction of the heart. Allow the oils to penetrate the skin. With high-quality natural oils, it doesn't take more than a couple of minutes to sink in. Smooth, touchable skin is just an added benefit to this time-honored technique.

In ancient Egypt, both men and women in all classes of society used body oiling. They saw that it was an effective way to maintain youth, vitality, and soft skin that would otherwise be dry and leathery in the hot desert sun.

Facial *Oiling*

We have a misguided understanding that applying oil to the face causes acne, blackheads, and breakouts. This simply isn't true. I've been cleansing, moisturizing, and exfoliating my face with carrier oils and essential oils for 15 years and simply love the luster of my skin. No acne, blackheads, or breakouts. Just radiant health!

Modern-day conventional soaps disrupt the endocrine, reproductive, digestion, and mental systems. They often contain cancer-causing sodium laurel sulphate, which creates bubbles or ethyl alcohol that strip the skin of valuable and necessary natural oils. In an effort to establish equanimity, our bodies need to recreate lost oils for normal skin balance once they have been removed. Cleansing the face with soap can lead to dry, excessively oily, or acne-prone skin, or premature wrinkles. Ditch the sudsy bar or liquid chemical "soap" and go Egyptian. Healing oils are where it's at.

Oils harmonize unbalanced skin, provide elasticity and tone, and even help remove the appearance of fine lines. I'm positively in love with jojoba for the face and body. Jojoba is an outstanding liquid wax that's one molecule away from skin sebum. (Sebum is an oily or waxy matter, excreted from that skin than makes it dewy and youthful. It lubricates and waterproofs the skin and hair of mammals.) Jojoba is incredibly stable and is preferable to sesame oil or apricot seed oil, as it has a long shelf life that maintains its potency and medicinal qualities for years. Our bodies naturally and authentically understand jojoba.

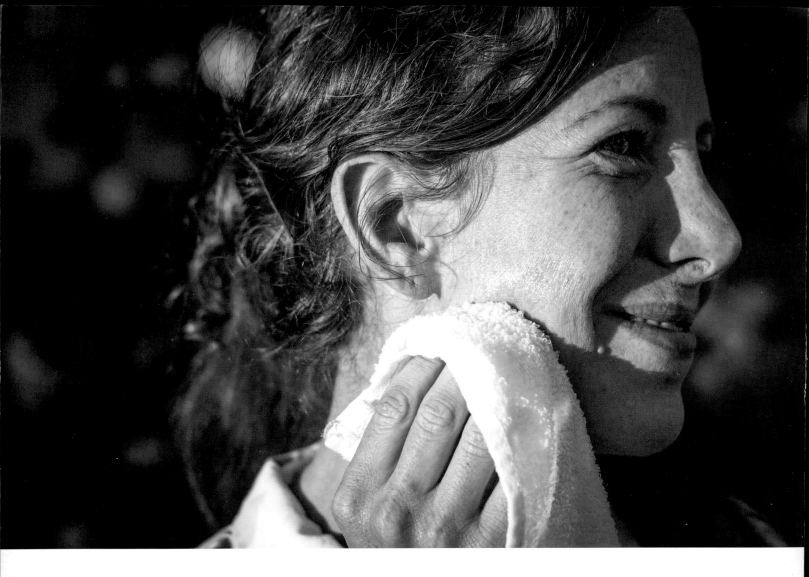

To cleanse the face, simply moisten it with either water or, to pamper yourself more luxuriously, use rose hydrosol. Add a small amount of oil to the face. Massage it into the face and neck in circular motions. Use a clean towel or hemp cloth to remove the oil and exfoliate the face in circular motions. Another method is to moisten the edge of a towel. Apply the oil directly to the moistened towel and then cleanse and exfoliate the face in one easy step. To finish and moisturize, add a few more drops of jojoba or another carrier oil. You can also easily remove eye makeup by applying oil to a damp cotton swab and wiping it over the eye until it's clean. Beauty never felt so good.

Oiling on a daily basis will improve skin elasticity and moisturize the skin, and it's a beautiful act of self-love. Use the time to state your self-love mantras loud and be proud. You are a flower with the

aromatherapy for sensual living *bewitching beauty rituals*

softest and most beautiful petals. Put that loving intention into every stroke and see how life trans-forms with your potent self-love. Massage, body oiling, and touch techniques are incredibly healthy for mind, body, spirit, and — most of all — heart.

You can create your own touch practices and improve the vitality of your health even if without a lover. In fact, learning to touch ourselves in loving, caring, and conscious ways can be even more powerful and healing than the touch of another.

Facial *Steams*

Facial steaming hydrates the skin during the long cold months of winter, removes blackheads and impurities, and adds a much appreciated pinch of luxury. One of my favorite ways to facial steam is to use hydrosols as the base in place of plain water. Hydrosols are the aromatic waters left over after the

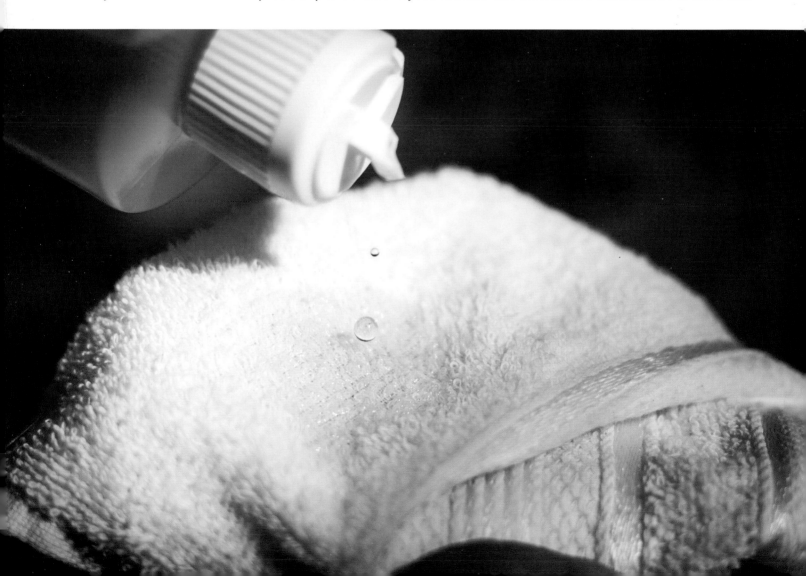

steam distillation process and are prized for their medicinal, aromatic, and nutritive qualities. When you use them for facial steams, you're imparting the pure, homeopathic versions of rose otto, neroli, lavender, or ylang ylang directly into the skin in a gentle yet highly effective way. Another benefit is that our lungs are treated to an aromatic steam bath, as hydrosols are powerful and prized liquid libations that promote health and vitality at the cellular level through the respiratory and circulatory systems.

If you don't have hydrosols available, you can easily replace them with pure essential oils and spring water or distilled water. Chemically treated, chlorine- and fluoride-laden tap water isn't suitable for the face or body. When we steam the face, the pores open to detoxify and draw in moisture, like the lungs. In using spring water, we shield the face from heavy metals, chlorine, fluoride, and nerve toxins found in many municipal water supplies.

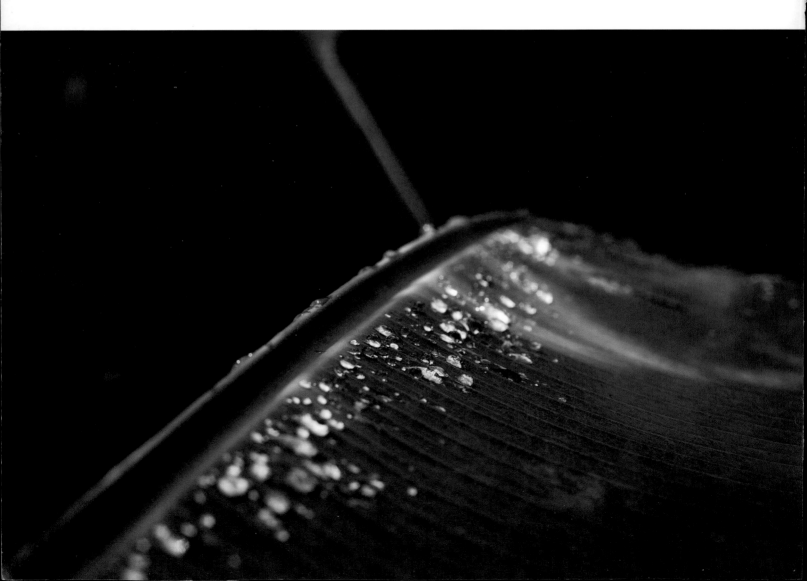

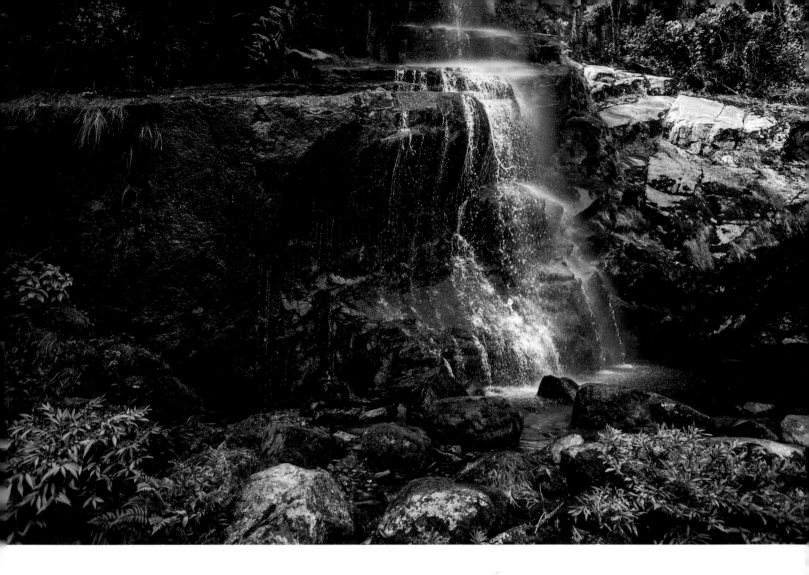

Add two to three drops of geranium, rose otto, frankincense, cape chamomile, sandalwood, neroli, lavender, or fenugreek to a large bowl of freshly boiled water. These oils are high in monoterpenes (chemical properties that regenerate, soften the skin, and smell absolutely divine). They're so gentle that they will not cause irritation or an unpleasant reaction.

Method

Place your face close to the bowl of aromatic water and allow the steam to mist your face. For a more concentrated treatment, place a towel over your head. Come up for air quite often because extreme heat over an extended period of time can cause burning and irritation to your delicate facial skin. Facial steaming should be a luxurious experience, not a torturous one. Use the steam treatment for ten to twenty minutes, followed with deep skin oiling. Feel free to gently exude blackheads and pimples after the facial steam because the pores will be open and pliable.

Facial steams are a fabulous way to go from scaly lizard skin to perfect peach in a matter of minutes, and you'll smell glorious too. It's about the way we treat and honor ourselves every day that will reflect love and care back into our lives.

Scrubs

At the beginning of my aromatherapy and healing career, I made custom salt and sugar scrubs for many of my clients. They were amazingly popular; everyone wanted to bathe and beautify in their own custom scent. It's a remarkably easy process and one that yields fantastic, curative results. I recommend using scrubs on the body rather than the face. Facial skin is simply too delicate for the coarse grains of either sugar or salt. To exfoliate the face, use a soft towel and the facial oiling method.

Salt will draw impurities out of the skin and replace lost minerals back into it, whereas sugar is a humectant, meaning that it will help to retain moisture, unlike salt. Additionally, they work beautifully to soften the skin. Always use either fine-grain Himalayan pink sea salt or organic cane sugar for best results.

Table salt contains bleach, ammonia, and anti-clumping agents to make it presentable to the average consumer. Conventional sugar is genetically modified and toxic. It is saturated with pesticides, herbicides, fungicides, bleach, and other toxins that shouldn't be put in or on your body. It's very important to use the highest quality organic ingredients in your path to total beauty.

Method

- Slowly melt one cup of coconut oil in a pot over gentle heat. Allow it to totally liquefy.
- Pour it into a glass bowl with four cups of salt or sugar in whatever combination that best suits you.

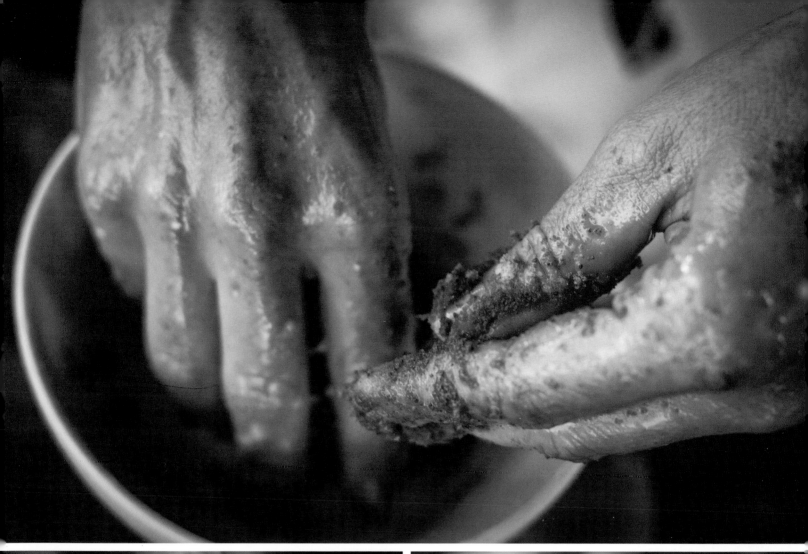
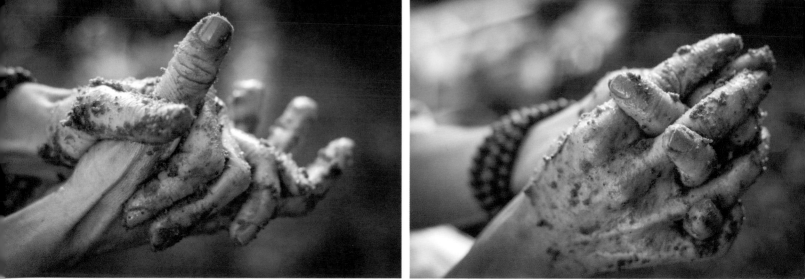

aromatherapy for sensual living   *bewitching beauty rituals*

- Mix well. Add more coconut oil to reach your desired level of creaminess. The blend should feel silky and cohesive rather than dry or overly oily. To amplify the pretty power, experiment by adding three tablespoons of aromatic herbs like rosemary, sage, mint, or thyme. You could also experiment with three tablespoons of dried violets, rosebuds, chamomile, jasmine, calendula, or lavender. Dried herbs and flowers give color and texture to your scrub creations.

- In a separate bottle, create a personalized blend using the blending principles outlined in the previous chapter. Half-fill a five-milliliter bottle (approximately 50 drops) with your choice of pure essential oils.

- Add your awesome essential oil blend to the salt or sugar mixture. Mix well.

- Store in an airtight glass jar away from light, heat, and air.

- Add one cup to a hot bath or use half a cup as an all-over body scrub.

Remember that herbs and flowers have aromatic and medicinal compounds. Consider the properties of the herbs when adding to your scrub blend. If you're making a sexy-time blend, the addition of sage (known for its ability to tame sexual energy, sharpen wits, clear unwanted energies, reduce breast milk, and relieve unwanted gas) might defeat the purpose. However, rosebuds, lavender, or jasmine flowers would definitely help enliven the sacred essence and make it so much more appealing.

An alternative base is pumice. It's a fine grain that's wonderful at sloughing off dead skin and can be used on the face. Remember that you're a fine flower who desires a gentle touch rather than a fierce pummel. Always exfoliate with care. You can find pumice at health food stores, herbal apothecaries, or higher quality pharmacies.

Use scrubs on the hands, feet, elbows, knees, buttocks, thighs, or anywhere that needs a little scrubbing action. The sugar combination is especially lovely to do with a partner. Don't be surprised if you find yourself licking your fingers while scrubbing in sweet satisfaction.

Scrubs are also very effective at breaking up the stagnation associated with cellulite. To treat stubborn cellulite, simply rub the scrub blend in circular and upward motions into dimpled points for five minutes every other day for at least three months. One of my favorite anti-cellulite scrubs is a fragrant combination of lemongrass, cypress, tangerine, lemon, and juniper berry. It's a powerful dimple-buster and smells oh so good.

Some luscious salt or sugar blends are:

- Black pepper, ginger, clove, and lemon: This is an excellent winter warming scrub, especially on the feet, hands, and ears.

- Rose otto, vanilla, lavender, magnolia flower, and fenugreek: This is a "let's get groovy tonight" blend. It's sexy, sweet, and bursting with flower power.

- Peppermint, tansy, lavender, and hay: This is a heavenly azure blend that's slightly cooling in nature and helps to soothe frazzled nerves.

- Lemongrass, black spruce, and cypress: This is a "rise and shine" blend. I used this blend for years in the morning to put a spring in my step.

- Marjoram, lavender, cape chamomile, and vanilla: This is a "sweet dreams" blend. The combination of these oils is deeply relaxing and calming to the central nervous system.

- Vetiver, Douglas fir, white cedar, mitti attar, and spikenard: This is a "buffed body for men" blend. I love when men smell of roots and trees. It's a loin-quivering combination.

In addition to scrubbing, cellulite can be diminished by avoiding greasy, fried, and rich foods; dairy products; and especially sugar (internally). Inappropriate dietary practices create and trap dampness in the body, which contributes to the appearance of unwanted cellulite. I suggest you do squats, take the stairs, or jump on your bike to strengthen muscles, improve circulation, and diminish unsightly dimpling.

Aloe *Vera Options*

I'm humbled by this simple plant for so many reasons. I once gave myself a nasty burn on my right hand by foolishly grabbing a hot pot. If I didn't know how to harness the power of plants, I would have been out of commission for at least four weeks. Who has that time?

Immediately upon receiving the burn, I used undiluted peppermint oil generously all over the hand in order to cool the fiery, throbbing heat. Once the initial heat left (after about fifteen minutes), I followed with undiluted lavender oil all over the burn every five minutes for one hour. I continued with a lavender/aloe combination until it looked like leathery but calm flesh. At this point, I was able to gently move my fingers without pain. I completed the treatment in five hours by applying aloe constantly and gently rubbing it into the wound. I was able to use my hands to teach later that day, and within 24 hours, there was no trace of the burn.

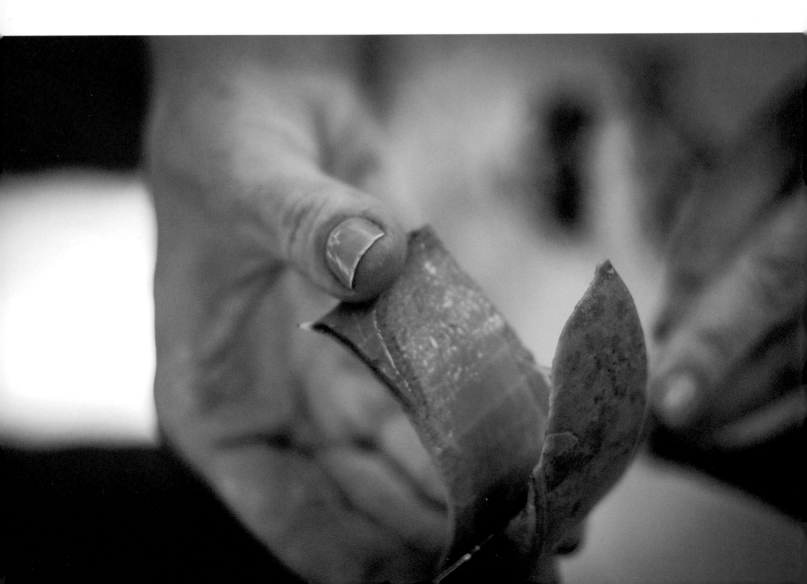

From that experience, I understood the connection between aloe and its skin regeneration properties. It's pure magic. I invite you to start using authentic raw aloe on your face every day. I assure that you'll see dramatic and restorative effects.

Aloe is remarkably easy to grow in your home. It just needs bright sunlight and minimal water. It will grow to the size of the pot, so keep replanting it to get big, juicy leaves. Once you've cut the leaves, store them in the refrigerator to maintain their freshness. Aloe can have a pungent smell when left out.

Aloe *Face Masks*

There are several different ways to use aloe along with essential oils for vibrant and amazing skin. Sometimes I skip all the fancy additions and simply mush the aloe over my face and allow it to soak in. It's incredibly refreshing and effectively keeps puffiness, fine lines, and spots away.

Mature/Dry *Skin*

½ to 1 inch of aloe vera
¼ of a ripe avocado
1 teaspoon of raw honey
1 drop of rose otto

Scrape out the aloe vera from its skin. Mash the avocado. Mix everything together and apply it to the skin for twenty minutes. Wash it off with warm water and apply jojoba. For extra benefit, spend a few moments in the sun to deepen the treatment.

Sensitive *or Sunburnt Skin*

½ to 1 inch of aloe vera
2 tablespoons of cucumber juice
1 tablespoon of raw goat yogurt

1 drop of peppermint oil
1 drop of lavender oil

Scrape out the aloe vera from its skin. Skin two inches of cucumber and pulse it in a food processor to obtain juice. Combine all of the ingredients in a small bowl and apply to the face or body. Leave it on for twenty minutes and rinse off. Repeat if necessary.

Acne-Prone *Skin*

½ to 1 inch of aloe vera
1 tablespoon of raw organic honey
1 drop of geranium or rosemary oil

Scrape out the aloe vera from its skin. Mix the remaining ingredients in a small bowl. Apply to your skin one to two times a week to achieve beautiful, clean, and clear skin.

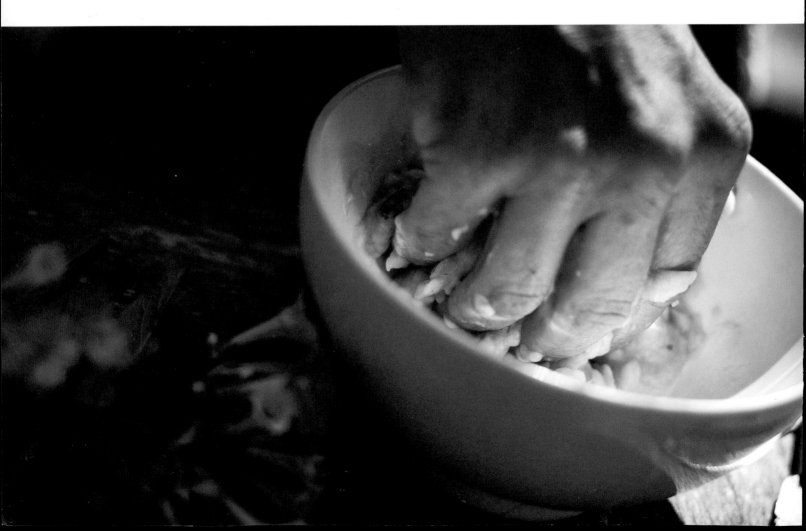

Deep *Hydration Mask*

½ to 1 inch of aloe vera
1 teaspoon of rose water
1 drop of frankincense oil

Scrape out the aloe vera and mash it up with the back of a fork. Mix it together with the other ingredients. Apply to face. Allow the blend to soak into the skin without washing it off. Once the blend is absorbed into the skin, finish with facial oiling.

Glowing *Skin Mask*

½ to 1 inch of aloe vera
1 teaspoon of honey
1 teaspoon of raw goat milk
1 drop of turmeric and fenugreek essential oil

Scrape out the aloe vera and mash it up. Add the remaining ingredients in a small bowl. Apply to the face for twenty minutes. Wash off with warm water and finish with facial oiling. Be aware that turmeric will stain your clothes and towels but give your face a healthy glow.

Honey *Mask*

Honey is a gift from the gods that tastes glorious and calms allergies; is an outstanding antibacterial agent; and is an effective way to care for broken skin. Anointing skin with honey will tone, exfoliate, and make skin look noticeably younger. Simply use one tablespoon of raw, organic honey along with one drop of essential oil. Mix well and apply to the face. Allow the blend to penetrate the face for a minimum of twenty minutes. Wash it off and anoint your skin with a carrier oil.

Other oils that are effective with honey are:

- Rose otto to improve elasticity and radiance (any left over makes a delicious edible love tonic)

- Lavender for general toning, relaxing, and freshening

- Geranium for deep healing and mature skin

- Sandalwood for fine lines, wrinkles, scars, and blackheads

- Frankincense to improve the radiance of the skin

- Cape chamomile for deep moisturization and restoration of the skin

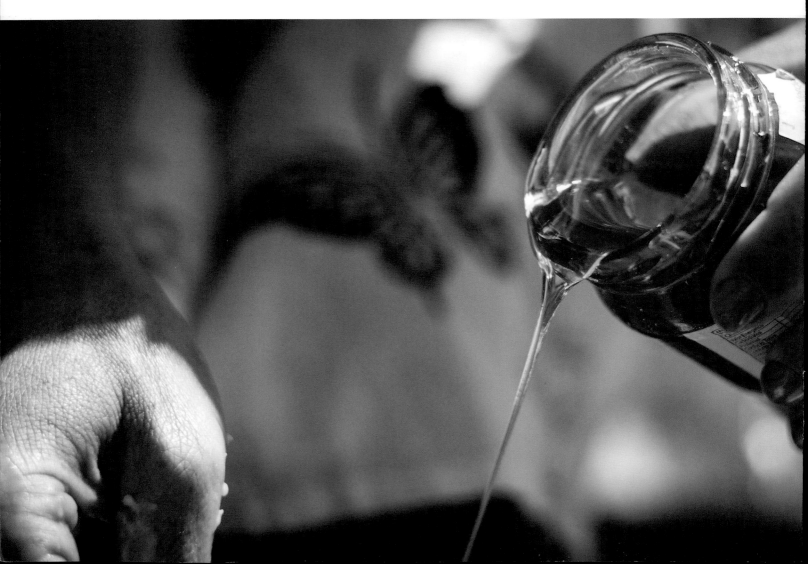

Clay *Masks and Muds*

Our earth is immensely giving and provides us with everything we need to be the beautiful, sensual creatures we're intended to be. There are a variety of clays to nourish and cleanse the skin on the face and body.

- **Green clay** helps to draw toxins and can calm inflammations. It's particularly good for acne.

- **White clay** soothes and softens the skin and is suitable for all skin types. This is the gentlest and most refined clay.

- **Red clay** is suitable for dry and sensitive skins.

- **Pink clay** is particularly useful for toning dull, tired, or devitalized skin. It also has excellent cleansing properties.

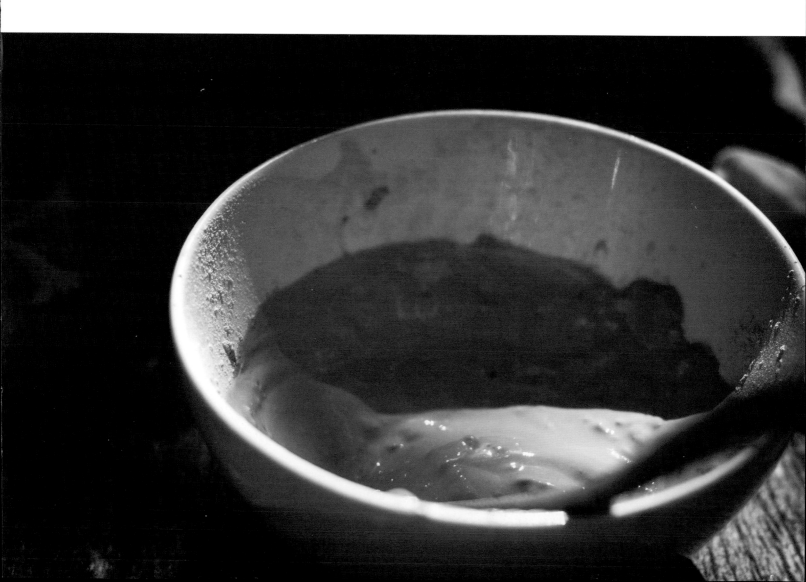

- **Bentonite clay** draws toxins from beneath the skin and is very effective at taming an acne breakout.

Combining clay masks with essential oils increases the effectiveness of the clays by gently pulling out impurities, nourishing the skin, and reducing fine lines.

Another option for brilliant beauty is to use mud masks. Muds tend to be more expensive than clay but have many benefits. Muds have a higher mineral content than clays, making them more nutritious to the skin. There is no mixing involved (except with the addition of essential oils). They detoxify and cleanse more deeply than clays and are considerably more moisturizing. Lastly, they are beneficial for most skin types, thus taking the guesswork out of which clay to use.

These blends can be used with either muds or clays. Use a maximum of five drops.

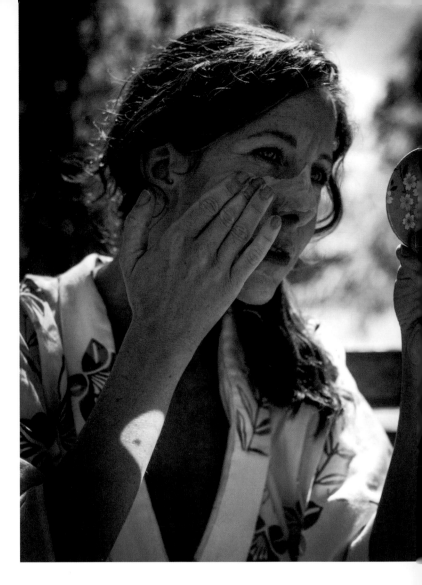

- Option 1 for mature or dry skin: cape chamomile, lavender, and sandalwood

- Option 2 for mature or dry skin: rose otto, frankincense, immortelle, and lavender

- Mature, acne-prone, or dull skin: neroli, geranium, and lemon

- Dry or inflamed skin: marjoram, lavender, and petitgrain

- Inflamed skin: cape chamomile, neroli, and lavender

aromatherapy for sensual living *bewitching beauty rituals*

Dry *Brushing*

Dry brushing is an ancient and effective technique to move lymph fluid around the body. The lymph is a clear watery fluid that detoxifies and carries pathogens out of the body. Unlike the venous system, the lymph system doesn't have a pumping mechanism to circulate it. We need to do hot/cold plunges, jumping exercises, or dry brushing to keep this vital system moving and grooving. When your lymph nodes are swollen, your body is working overtime to remove the bacteria, pathogens, or viruses.

Using a dry brush with essential oils is a one-two punch of vitality, energy, and soft, glowing skin. You can buy dry brushes at any health food store and many pharmacies.

Method

- Place one drop of a lymph essential oil blend in the palm of your hand.

- Rub your hands together and then rub the dry brush with your hands to anoint the bristles.

- Start by tapping your main lymph nodes under your armpits, on the stomach and groin, behind the knees, and on the inner ankles.

- Place the bristles of the brush on the tops of the feet and brush up your body. Always brush in the direction of your heart. Be sure to cover all parts of your body, including the stomach, buttocks, and back. There are many lymph nodes in the stomach area.

- Dry brush for two to five minutes every day.

One of the additional benefits of dry brushing is that it acts in place of coffee to give you your morning jolt. You'll feel alert and ready immediately without the jittery rush. Dry brushing supports healthy living, circulation, and detoxification pathways in the body. And it won't give you coffee breath or stained teeth.

For lymph blends, use one to two drops on the brush per day. For these formulas, I recommend you make a whole body to have it ready to go when you are potentially rushed in the morning.

Lymph *Brush Blends*

- Cypress, black spruce, red cedar, white cedar, sage

- Zinziba, lemongrass, rosemary, thyme linalool

- Juniper berry, fennel, eucalyptus, lemon

- Rosemary, lime, Douglas fir, laurel

- Cinnamon, cardamom, rose absolute, vanilla (This is also a very sexy blend.)

Your *Glorious Tresses*

"I am caught in this curling energy, your hair. Whoever is calm and sensible is insane." – Rumi

A woman's hair is her crown. She can adorn it with flowers, create dramatic styles, or use it to slyly hide from the world. Locks evoke passion with a dramatic flick, a twirl on a finger, or a toss at just the right time. Never underestimate your ability to tease and charm with your hair.

Hair is also a clear indication of your health. If you are losing your hair, graying, have fine hair, or hair that easily breaks, there's so much you can do. My sweet flower, you never need to suffer with limp locks.

I have basic protocols I use for my clients who are losing their hair or want to amplify their hair to gorgeous bombshell levels.

- Massage five drops of rosemary essential oil into the scalp along with half a teaspoon of coconut oil every day. Rosemary has a long-standing reputation of helping hair to grow and thicken. It also effectively wards off mental fatigue and boosts memory retention. Coconut oil has long been used to moisturize and stimulate hair follicles. It is also a handy-dandy sexual stimulant too.

- Fo ti (he sho wu) is a Chinese adaptogen herb that's revered for its ability to restore and regrow hair. I use a teaspoon of this herb every day in my morning smoothie. You can buy it at Chinese supermarkets, pharmacies, or better quality health food stores. It takes quite a few months of regular use, but your hair will come back with flowing and healthy vitality.

- Reduce your stress level. If you're frazzled, you'll lose vitality and hair luminosity. Take a yoga class, breathe deeply, and seek beauty in nature. Additionally, use adaptogen herbs such as rhodiola, schizandra berry, or cordycepts to help mitigate stress patterns and support your kidneys and adrenals.

- Aloe vera gel is very effective at helping promote hair growth. Scrape out the gel from thick leaves and apply it to the hair for twenty minutes. Cover your hair from root to tip. Repeat once a week or use it as a daily conditioner

- Eat good fats (including ghee, coconut oil, butter, organic olive oil, and chia seeds) and green leafy vegetables. All of these help to restore healthy vitality to skin, hair, and nails.

- Brahmi oil or powder is a holy oil in India that's used for hair health, to boost neurological function (it's applied to children with autism), and to help with sleep disorders. Massage a small amount into the scalp every day. It smells delicious, too. I recently found Brahmi powder that can easily be added to morning smoothies.

- Once you've stabilized your hair, then you can start getting into some luscious practices that will effectively boost shine and buoyancy while unleashing the sex siren in your hair.

Hair Treatments

Hot Oil

Hot oil treatments are a very effective way to deeply emolliate the hair. Start with two tablespoons of coconut oil, warmed slightly on the stove (never use a microwave to heat oils), along with up to six to eight drops from the oil blends listed below. Apply to your hair from root to tip. Deeply massage your head with firm, directed pressure. This is a sinfully pleasurable activity to do with a partner. Spend a few moments pulling your hair to bring blood and circulation to the scalp. It feels amazing and will give you shinier hair. Leave the treatment on for at least thirty minutes and up to eight hours, preferably while covered. Wash out with mild, natural shampoo and finish with conditioner.

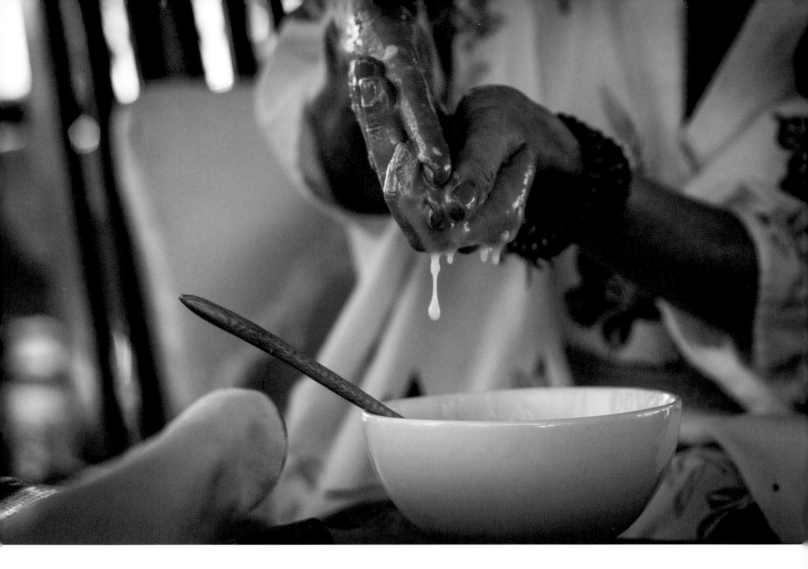

Some exotic, outstanding hair essential oil blends are:

- Rosemary, basil, lavender

- Ylang ylang, bergamot, clove

- Cardamom, vanilla, immortelle

- Jasmine, hay, blood orange, vanilla

- Lemongrass, lemon, lavender, rosemary

aromatherapy for sensual living *bewitching beauty rituals*

Raw *Coconut Water Hair Treatment*

Applying raw coconut water to the hair is a fantastic way to deeply moisturize and condition. My favorite way is to apply it to the hair, massage it in deeply, and then comb through. Allow it to dry completely, preferably in the sun. Wash the coconut water out a few hours later. You'll find your hair is full of body, bounce, and shine. Isn't that what all sensual lovers are seeking? Adding essential oils to hair blends will only deepen the treatment.

Clean *Hair Treatment*

Even with the most valiant of efforts to keep our hair shiny and luminous, sometimes our locks fall flat. Pollution, chemical hair products, dirt, and grime all make our locks less lovely. Apple cider vinegar deeply cleanses the hair without stripping it of valuable oils and removes unsightly dandruff.

Apple cider vinegar is an alkaline vinegar, so it will clean your hair without harm. It's effective at toning skin, supporting complete digestion, detoxifying the liver, getting rid of candida, and so much more. To clean your hair, simply mix half a cup of apple cider vinegar with half a cup of warm water. Wet your hair and slowly pour the mixture over your head, saturating the entire head with the combination. Massage deeply for three to five minutes. Rinse out the mixture and continue with regular shampoo and conditioner. It's instant bounce and shine.

You can amplify the cleaning action with these essential oils: lemon, peppermint, tea tree, rosemary, basil, lemongrass, white spruce, cypress, juniper berry, and bergamot.

Dry *Hair*

I naturally have curly hair that's susceptible to dryness and parches in the sun while I luxuriate around pools and dip in lakes in the summer. In the winter, it withers due to a lack of moisture and radiant heat. This amounts to limp locks and potentially split ends.

One of my favorite ways to super-hydrate my hair and tame the unfriendly frizz is to use natural butters. Butters are thick, deeply emollient treasures. Apply a small amount to the tips of hair and watch curls form into bouncy perfection. You can also use butters as a pre-shampoo hair treatment. Simply allow a quarter-sized amount of butter to melt in your hand and apply it to your hair from root to tip. Massage and leave it in for at least twenty minutes or even overnight. Wash out with regular shampoo and conditioner. Do this treatment every seven to fourteen days for gorgeous hair.

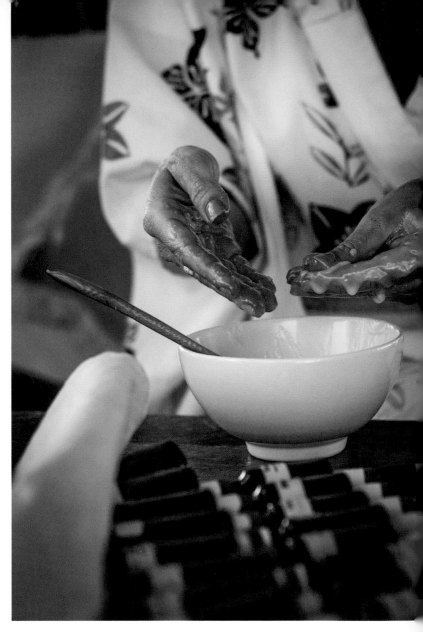

Luscious *Lover Body Butter*

- Add ⅔ cup cacao butter, ⅓ cup shea butter, ⅓ cup coconut oil and a generous splash of jojoba into a double boiler.

- Use the lowest heat possible that allows the oils to melt down entirely.

- Remove from heat and add your choice of essential oils, stirring gently.

- Pour into a clean, sterilized jar and place in the freezer on an even surface overnight.

- Take out of the freezer. Allow the mixture to come to room temperature. Use anywhere you could use a little extra moisture in your life.

This blend can also be used for a natural love lube, skin moisturizer, furniture polish, hair de-frizzer, and lip balm. I find it endlessly sexy to apply the same scented butters I use in the bedroom to moisturize my lips or tame flyaway hair. It's a not-so-innocent reminder of previous pursuits.

aromatherapy for sensual living *bewitching beauty rituals*

Some beautiful butter combinations are:

- Cinnamon, vanilla, tangerine

- Lavender, rose otto, sandalwood

- Cape chamomile, immortelle, fenugreek

- Cardamom, carnation, clove

- Tuberose, hay, lemon

- Spikenard, geranium, bergamot

Hand *and Foot Treatments*

Kiss your hands, love the lines, celebrate the spots; you've earned them. There's something so beautiful and honestly genuine about a woman with experience. There are, however, various ways that we can care for the skin of our hands to help them stay supple and healthy on a deep level. One of my favorite hand treatments is a two-step process: a sugar scrub followed by a hot oil infusion.

Wrapping hands with warm oils is particularly effective for those with osteoarthritis or rheumatoid arthritis, as both are inflammatory conditions. While essential oils can reduce inflammation and increase circulation, essential oils won't rebuild cartilage. There are many supplements and herbs that can additionally help with this condition. That being said, applying warm oils to hands can be a tremendously healing and pain-reducing protocol. It's also totally luxurious.

Melt two tablespoon of coconut oil with one teaspoon of jojoba oil over a double boiler on a mellow heat. Add five to ten drops of a softening hand oil blend to the mix. Apply the warmed blend to your hands and/or feet. Cover your hands or feet with wool socks and allow the oils to penetrate your skin for a minimum of twenty minutes to overnight. Wipe the remainder of the oil off with a cloth.

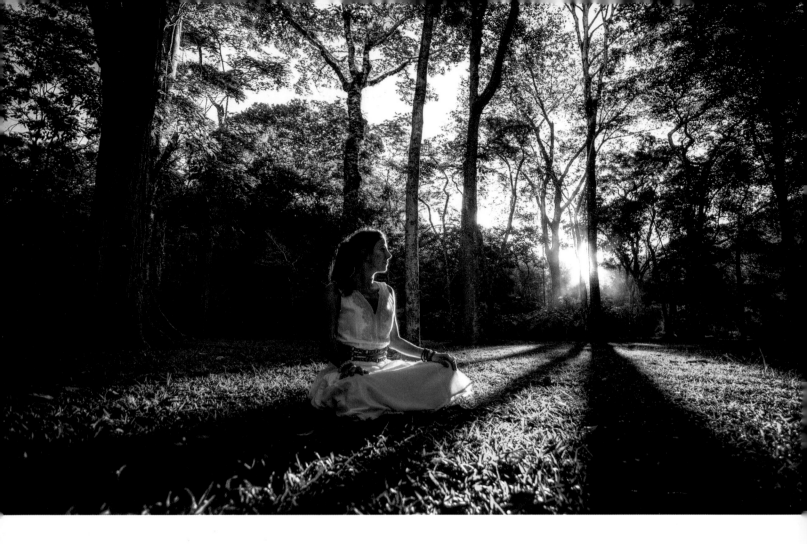

Some of my favorite hand blends are:

- Marjoram, black pepper, sandalwood

- Clove, peppermint, vetiver

- Lemon, lavender, ginger

- Cinnamon, grapefruit, immortelle

- Thyme linalool, eucalyptus, marjoram

- Rose otto, fenugreek, fennel

- Juniper berry, cypress, sandalwood

- Lavender, ylang ylang, lemon

aromatherapy for sensual living *bewitching beauty rituals*

Deepening *Sensuality: How to Make Hydrosols*

Hydrosols are the aromatic and medicinal waters that remain after the steam distillation process. You can easily make hydrosols with a homemade still. It's a bit of witchy magic and a great way to experiment with plants. Hydrosols are wonderfully versatile and can be used to anoint your face; to cleanse and heal; as a vaginal douche; or even to flavor foods and drinks.

- Start with a large non-metal pot (clear glass is preferred) with a snug-fitting lid so vapor or volatile oils aren't lost when the water is boiling.

- Place a one- to two-inch clean stone or brick into the glass pot. The stone should be large enough to support the weight of a heat-resistant bowl.

- Select your choice of aromatic herbs or flowers, such as petals from three dozen organic roses, three cups of chamomile flowers, or fourteen stems of rosemary or lavender. If you're using roses, pluck the heads from the stems and carefully separate the petals, touching them as little as possible.

- Add the plant material to the bottom of the pot, making sure to keep the surface of the stone or double boiler free to hold the glass bowl.

- Use just enough spring or distilled water to cover the herbs. Put the glass bowl on top of the stone.

- Take the lid of the pot and turn it upside down on top of the pot so the curved handle is directly above the glass bowl.

- Bring the water to a gentle simmer (be sure not to boil the water). Reduce the heat to medium low.

- Once you've turned down the heat, place a sealed bag of ice on top of the inverted lid. Make sure that there are no steam holes on the lid as it will melt the plastic and contaminate the hydrosol. The ice causes the hot water to condense and then fall directly into the glass bowl receptacle, which catches the hydrosol.

- Allow the hydrosol to collect in the bowl for a maximum of eight hours. Continue to check the hydrosol to ensure that the heat isn't too high or that the receptacle bowl isn't overflowing. Discard the plant material once the water has entirely evaporated.

- Pour all contents of the glass bowl into a heat-resistant sterilized jar or bottle. Store in a cool, dark place. If done properly, the hydrosol will be potent for six months to a year.

Your radiating beauty is a gift to the world. When you sparkle and shine, you reflect the true beauty of the divine through you and inspire others to do the same. It's your witchy woman beauty power. Consider what more you can do to help yourself bloom into the vivacious and luscious lily that you are.

Love yourself and your body, dimples and all. When we take time every day to love ourselves, we create positive ripples in the rest of our lives and in all of our relationships. When we do, we're in a better position to be met in love, stand up for ourselves, feel confident in our bodies, and sway with ease. Self-love is the droplet that starts a tidal wave of good and positive things in your life. Love it all.

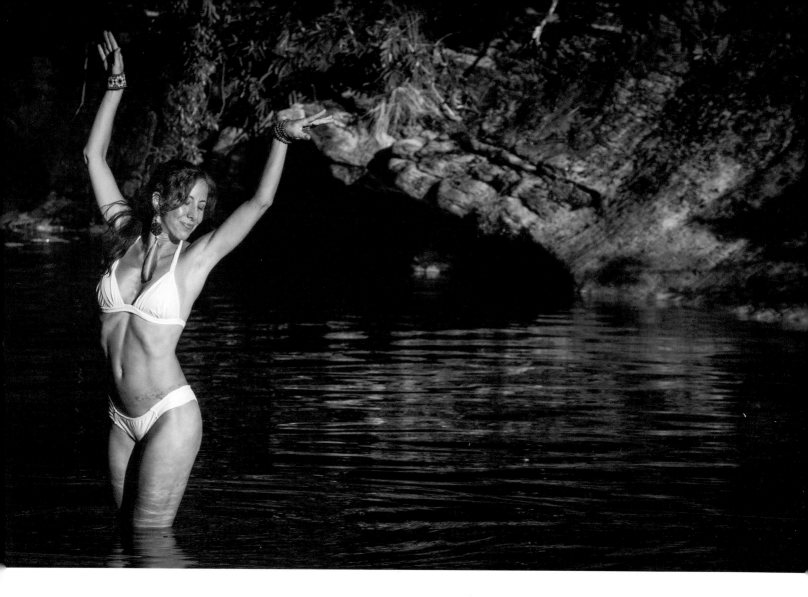

Zen States of Sensuality

Sensuality is alluring. It's commanding our innate, life-giving power that we express between our legs and through our hearts and minds. Women who own it — themselves, their space and their beauty — are sparkling diamonds.

Another type of sensuality is to simply feel good in our own bodies, within our personal spaces; quiet, whole, simple, peaceful, and in love with life and ourselves. It's the beauty that comes when no one is watching. Sensuality can be quiet rather than imposing and remain ever so evocative.

I've included several ways to utilize essential oils to increase your peace and allow you to be luminous in your natural beauty. Essential oils provide the magic carpet to glide you into the garden of love in their holy perfection.

Bathing

When I bathe with essential oils, I connect with my aroma oil friends to receive their deep healing information directly into my body, lymph, and limbic system. It's deeply therapeutic, nurturing, and fortifying to the mind, body, and soul.

For baths, use five to ten drops of oil and a combination of sea salt, Epsom salt, baking soda, organic sugar, coconut oil, and/or jojoba oil. Sometimes if I'm looking to heal my heart, solve a difficult emotional problem, or simply unwind, I forgo any additions or combinations and just use a singular essential oil. It's quiet time for me to tune into one frequency. This speaks to the power of plants and the myriad of information they impart.

In terms of erotic proclivities, I think that getting into a steamy bath with your sweetheart is just about one of the most wonderful things imaginable; it's quiet, naked, healing time to connect and cuddle.

For a sensual baths, I recommend using coconut oil to deeply emolliate the skin, sea salt to detoxify, and Dr. Bronner's Castile soap to make blissful bubbles. Any combination of euphoric oils would work well here (a maximum of ten drops). If you are bathing with a man or someone who leans toward masculine scents, I recommend using some of the heavier base notes so he/she is not put off by a bouquet of sweet-smelling flowers, unless he/she is into that kind of thing.

Some wonderful bathing blends for you and your lover are:

- Sandalwood, carnation, lavender

- Vanilla, tangerine, geranium

- Rose absolute, white cedar, lemon

- Jasmine, lavender, lime

- Vetiver, cypress, Douglas fir

- Cape chamomile, black pepper, frankincense

- Fenugreek, lemon, vanilla

- Ginger, grapefruit, laurel

- White cedar, patchouli, palo santo

- Ylang ylang, lavender, hay

Experiment and play. To create a deeply romantic experience, I recommend that you and your lover create a sacred blend together that encapsulates the union and devotion you share. Infuse it with the most profound love. Slowly drop it into the bath, and then get wet and wild together. Don't forget the bubbles. Complete the experience with mutual, long, and languid body oiling. It might just be the sweetest, most connected bliss.

Sauna

I never need to be convinced to sauna. Being warm, wet, and naked is one of my favorite things. Scandalous memories aside, saunas are also deeply healing. They are incredibly effective in detoxing organs and blood on a deep level. They improve circulation, clear the skin and lungs of impurities, detox heavy metals and, most importantly, are a total bliss trip for the mind and body. Saunas are the perfect vehicle to help us come into that quiet, peaceful, and sensual calm that we all crave. It's the true zen state of sensuality. This coveted state exists only if you give yourself the time and space to open to it. Saunas are quantifiably more effective when combined with the healing powers of essential oils.

There are several ways to use essential oils in the sauna to make the experience that much more healing and enticing.

- Apply essential oils directly onto the hot stones to send the antimicrobial, antiviral, anti-fungal, and erotic properties directly into the skin and lungs.

- Add essential oils to a bucket of water and cup the aromatic water on the hot stones. Just be sure that the sauna heater is designed for steam.

- Moisten a washcloth dosed with essential oils. Gently scrub the skin with the cloth so the oil goes directly into the bloodstream through the open pores and sloughs off the dead skin. This process makes for noticeably soft and touchable skin and a healthier constitution.

- Moisten a second cloth with water and essential oils. Cover the face and mouth with the cloth and breathe warm, wet, medicinal air. Rosemary, cypress, juniper berry, eucalyptus, Douglas fir, red cedar, and frankincense are excellent oils for this method as these oils are very effective for those with lung conditions. The addition of lavender, geranium, rose otto, or frankincense will tame certain skin conditions, though any essential oils in saunas will support and fortify the lungs and improve overall health.

Meditation

Aromatic smoke has been used in churches, temples, and ceremonies since the beginning of time to help people enter into a meditational, devotional place. While I sometimes use smoke for my meditations, more often I place a single drop of oil on a tissue and tuck it in my shirt for the duration of my practice. In doing so, my meditations are easier and deeper. I slip into the dreamy bliss place with considerably less resistance.

Essential oil meditations are a perfect way to cool any pre-date jitters, ground your energy, and focus your intent for the evening. Ask your lover to join your aroma meditation before indulging in the sacred act. It's a beautiful way to tune into each other's subtle frequencies and become present for each other. Meditations and bedroom romps are greatly enhanced by the using one of the more erotic base notes. It will help you maintain a focused calm while also revving your engines. Isn't sexy calm confidence the exact thing we're going for? It is the foundation of *Sensual Living*.

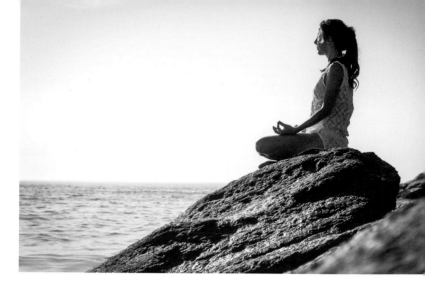

To meditate, I recommend simply sitting down in a comfortable, cross-legged position on a cushion with knees supported or lying down with a straight spine. Close your eyes and focus on the inward and outward exhalations of your breath. Notice when your mind carries you off into another direction. Quietly and gently bring your mind back by simply breathing. Keep it light and aim to meditate for twenty to thirty minutes.

Some of my favorite oils for seductive aroma meditations are frankincense, sandalwood, vetiver, jasmine, ylang ylang, geranium, rose absolute, and patchouli.

To create the conditions for a blissful night's sleep try lavender, cape chamomile, marjoram, or sandalwood. These oils have deeply sedating properties and will relax the mind and body.

Sunbathing

Who doesn't feel positively blissed out while lounging on the beach? It is by far one of my favorite sensual pastimes. It's a shocker for many that I don't use traditional sunscreen. Instead, I use a blend of essential oils in a base of seabuckthorn, red raspberry leaf, and jojoba to gently allow the healing rays of the sun into my skin without burning (for the appropriate length of time).

There are many benefits to sunbathing in moderation, including healing skin tissue (in the cases of burns, fungal infections, eczema, and psoriasis) and strengthening bones. The sun is a powerful antidepressant. It's an effective way to support the immune system and increase blood production. The sun has a great effect on stamina, fitness, and muscular development. I have a whole-hearted love-on for the sun's glorious, warming rays.

If you're using essential oils in the sun, be sure to not use oils from the citrus family such as tangerine, lemon, grapefruit, lime, or blood orange, as these oils are phototoxic. They'll make you more susceptible to penetrating sun rays and, potentially, a bad burn.

My favorite way to use essential oils is to expose my spine for up to forty-five minutes to the sun before noon. I anoint my front column with diluted essential oils and allow my back exposure to the sun. The result is harmonious and healing. The oils that I like to use for sun worship are geranium, lavender, cape chamomile, tansy, sandalwood, tarragon, magnolia blossom, and ginger lily.

Going *Blind to Enhance our Senses*

When we restrict one sense, our other senses (and pleasure buttons) come to life. These exercises are intended to enhance your individual senses for the purpose of becoming more sensual, present, at peace, and closer to the divine. Additionally, "going blind" is a fantastic and delightfully pleasurable activity to do with your love friend. There is an endless amount to discover.

Blind *Smelling*

We make a lot of assumptions based on what we've been told about specific oils and their properties. This exercise encourages you to develop your own essential oil vocabulary so that you'll understand how to use oils for your individual purposes.

Cover up the label of essential oil bottles so you can't see their names. Smell the oil using three deep breaths. Take note of where the oil goes in your body. Become aware of any thoughts, feelings, memories, or emotions that come up. Discern if the oil is a top, middle, base, or euphoric note based on how you feel when you smell it. Try to guess the name of the oil. Start an aromatic diary to better understand the oils and their individual uses that are unique to you. I love this exercise because you can learn so much about the oils and their properties by using only your nose as a guide.

Blind *Touching*

Our fingertips have dense receptors that come alive when sight is restricted. To enhance this sense, collect a variety of objects with unique and varied textures. With your eyes covered, slowly touch the objects. Allow the objects to touch your fingers, inner thigh, lips, feet, inner arm, and face. Another way to blind touch is to let your fingers to trace over your lover's body. Explore curves and crevices of your beloved in a unique, seductive way. It's yours to discover. Let the experience evoke pleasure through your whole body. Touch is so provocative.

Blind *Tasting*

Food can be gloriously sexy. In the Tangerine Temptation section, we explored the pleasure of eating slowly and with full sensual awareness. This time, have your lover prepare small, bite-sized portions of raw chocolate, pineapple, mango, raspberries, or other fruits. Have him/her blindfold you and slowly feed you different foods. Take time to experience the different texture, taste and sweetness. You may have an entirely different reaction to the food once your sight is restricted. As an added benefit, add a drop of essential oil. There's some juicy magic when fruit and edible essential oils commingle. It's medicinal, too.

Deepening *Sensuality: Become the Rose*

One of the best ways to comprehend the energy, knowledge, and divinity of flowers is this simple, powerful meditation. It will heighten your awareness of the plant kingdom and some say that it calms anxiousness and improves psychic ability. The more detail you can use in your meditation, the more powerful it will be. Take at least ten minutes and three cycles to complete this meditation.

In your mind's eye, imagine a tiny rose seed germinating in the ground. Notice as it sends its little hairy roots into the soil while simultaneously using all of its energy to burst forth from the earth. The small, detailed, green leaves slowly unfurl as the stalk continues to shoot upward toward the sky. Imagine the rose head slowly appearing at the top of the stalk, tightly compacted into a tiny green bulb. It is both excited and nervous. Leisurely allow the green bulb to unfurl to reveal the rich red blossom tucked into itself. It's the moment the rose has worked so hard to achieve. Feel the petals directing their energy outward, allowing them to part and the flower to bloom. Observe the rich red color as it brightens and deepens to spreads itself out. Note the fullness of the blossom and infinite petals of the rose. God exists in flowers. Breathe in the unique aroma and the gorgeous complexities of the flower. Take it in fully. Let it thrill you and take your breath away. Feel the fullness and exquisite beauty course through your whole body, into every cell. Become the flower. Breathe for a moment in this bliss.

Now watch the rose petals wither slightly. See how the edges of the petals turn brown, turn in and, one by one, gently fall to the ground. Notice the rose hips in the center of the rose. Note their color, texture, size and shape. Aren't they so delicious? At the bottom of the stalk, observe the fallen petals as they decay and go back into the ground, providing essential nourishment for the soil. Feel the weight of your fallen petals on the ground. Watch the stalk lose its vitality and shrink as the energy descends back into the ground. Watch the leaves also curl in and fall. Note the quiet, earth-directed, descending

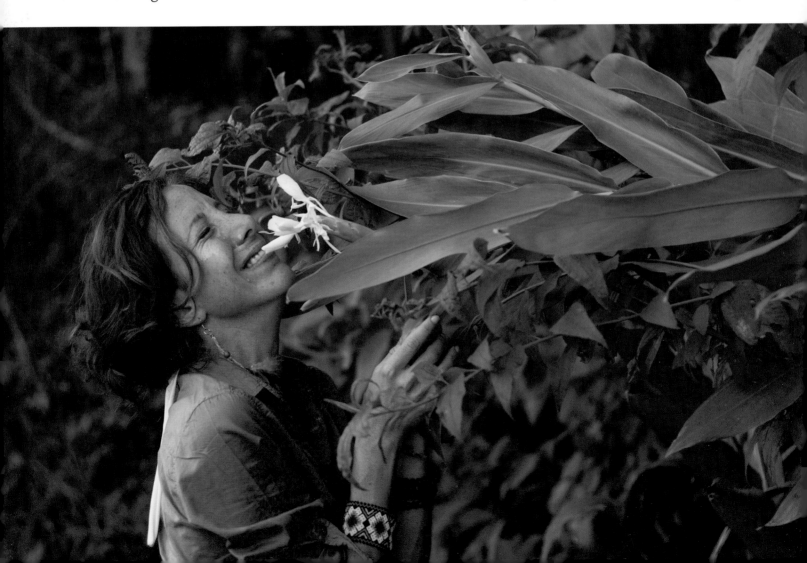

energy. Allow that feeling to circulate through your body. How do you feel? Note any emotion that comes up while the rose is in its dormancy. Sit with those emotions for a moment.

Continue the rose meditation, repeating the cycle three times. To enhance the meditation, anoint your nose and third eye with rose otto or rose absolute.

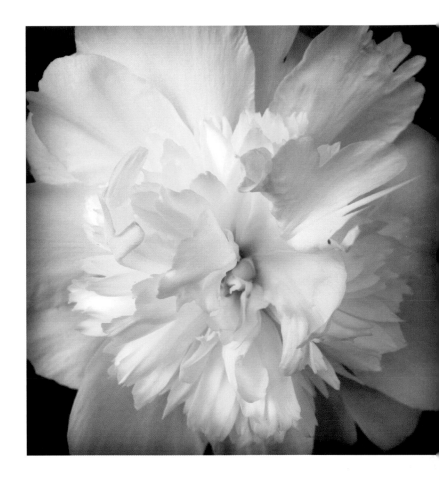

"**Pure** *Beauty" by Sônia Palhares*

I see the forest humid from the rain
A luminous green shines over the earth
And the rainbow, this king of beautiful colors
Such perfection, not an illusion

I see the flowers, such sublime beings
What exists more beautiful than a garden
And the fresh dewdrops on the rose
How beautiful is the flower

And I ask,
How to be the pure beauty of Love
And I ask,
How to be the pure beauty of Love

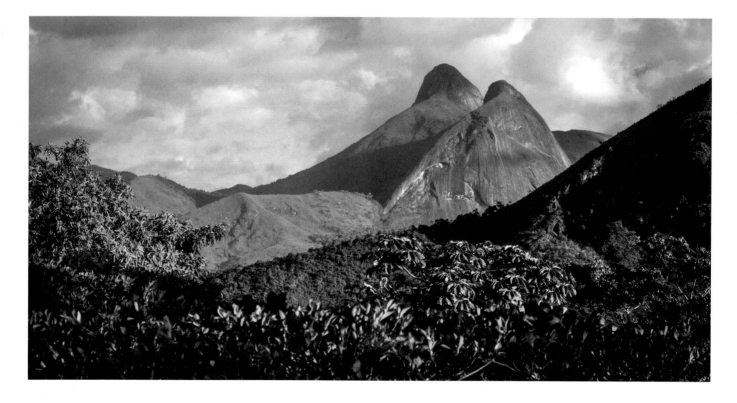

aromatherapy for sensual living *zen states of sensuality*

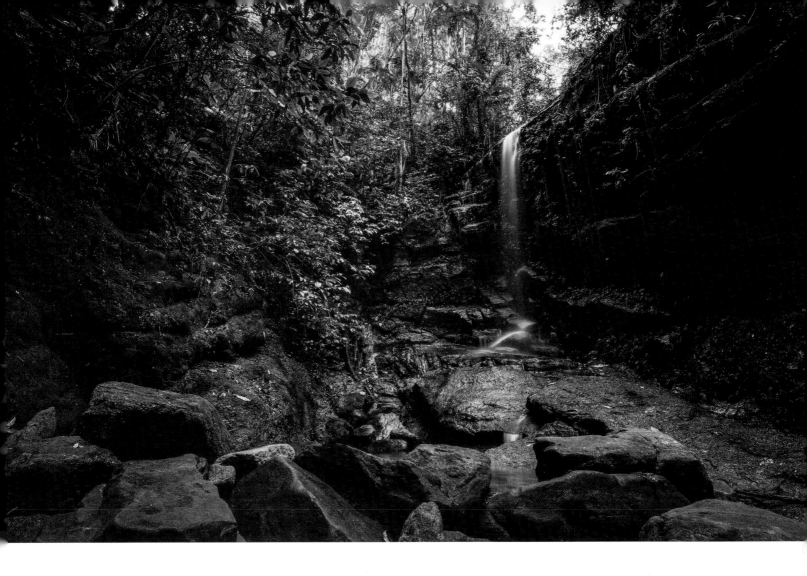

Steamy, Dreamy, Creamy: Enthralling Essential Oil Practices

Essential oils are an invitation for seduction and long, hot nights of play. Here are some of my favorite ways to use them to boost libido, deepen a connection with your sweetheart, and send your spirit to the cosmos. With aromatic sensuality, you're not just invoking smell but engaging all the senses to create the most delightful memories. Create a scene. Be creative. The connection between perfume and sex is ancient. There's a reason why it has stuck around for so long.

Here are some ways to deepen sensuality using essential oils:

- Add one drop of immortelle and one drop of cape chamomile together in a bowl with a tablespoon or so of raw honey. Mix it together. Take turns feeding each other the blend. Allow the blend to slowly melt on your tongue and let it roll all over the different taste centers before you swallow. Take time to track where the oils go in your body. That alone is a stimulating experience. Both of these essential oils are euphorics and will cause an exquisite, illicit reaction every time without exception.

  Other combinations are immortelle and tangerine; rose otto and lemon; sandalwood and lavender; vanilla, immortelle, and cape chamomile; neroli and vanilla; cinnamon and tangerine.

- Draw a bath with six drops of jasmine, four drops of lavender, and two drops of black pepper, along with sea salt and a tablespoon of coconut oil. This bath will draw out toxins, emolliate the skin, and infuse your cells with potent sexy-time oils. Bathing is a sacred practice that allows deep and connected time together. Commit to consciously connecting through your eyes. Make the bath a stress-free zone where the only purpose is to deepen your connection to each other and the love that you share. Exchange massages, wash each other's backs, and get pruned together. Couples who bathe together stay together and are happier when they use aromatic augmentations.

  Other bath time combinations are: ginger, grapefruit, and clove; osmanthus, bergamot, and vanilla; tangerine and vetiver; tuberose, lavender, and vanilla; immortelle and geranium; and jasmine, black pepper, and blood orange.

- Scent your mattress, pillowcase, or sheets with essential oils. I do this in hotels to clear other people's energy and feel more at home. Make sure that you're using clear, colorless oils so you don't stain your sheets.

  Some wonderful oils to use are osmanthus, neroli, lavender, cypress, rosemary, tuberose, Douglas fir, white fir, palo santo, and ylang ylang.

aromatherapy for sensual living *steamy, dreamy, creamy: enthralling essential oil practices*

- Rub essential oils between your hands and then through your hair. Who doesn't want to inhale beautiful-smelling hair? This method makes the aroma last for a long time and will combat any dirty-hair smell in between washes.

  Use any oil that you're attracted to for this exercise. Rosemary, cypress, black spruce, basil, and tangerine are great brain-boosting oils. I love using sandalwood and vanilla.

- Take one drop of essential oil in your mouth along with honey, chocolate, or coconut oil. Exchange aromatic kisses. Slowly blow aroma-infused caresses all over your lover's body. Be sure to blow on feet, the back of the neck, wrists, back of the knees, breasts, and ears. Blowing with different levels of force can be absolutely stimulating as the aroma is absorbed through the skin of your lover.

  Some excellent oils to use are cardamom, rose otto, vanilla, ginger, rose, geranium, cinnamon, allspice, fenugreek, cape chamomile, and immortelle.

I invite you to create the most luscious, exciting, dramatic scene to entice your lover. Be bold and confident in your practices. It's a sacred moment for you to share with someone special. Not everyone gets to see you naked with your heart racing, face flushed, and shuddering with desire. Use that power for good. It's your pretty petal power. Your intention and a little bit of planning will create lasting memories and a deep healing space.

Cleopatra, Queen of the Nile, was known for her love of essential oils and their power to evoke an erotic response. She would soak her sails in rose otto so that her scent would reach across the Mediterranean to her lover, Mark Antony, long before she arrived. She was a lady with style.

There are various ways to help create a stimulating environment. Here are some tips on setting the mood:

- Bring colorful pillows and soulful music into your love space.

- Turn your lights down low and light a variety of beeswax candles. Regular candles are petroleum-based and some people can be sensitive to the toxic fumes created by burning them. Beeswax candles are natural, smell great, and even help to remove dust from your love nest.

- Decant essential oils and carrier oils into wine or champagne glasses so pouring them on your lover feels that much more indulgent.

- As you anoint your lover's body, wrap him or her in the softest Pima cotton, heavy hemp, lovely linen, or richest silk. Soft fabrics on smooth skin enrich any experience.

- Watch the oils slowly drop out of the bottle in electrifying anticipation of things to come.

- Deeply breathe in the oils, both singularly and in combination, to invoke your lover. It will remind his/her limbic brain of a connection to the natural, erotic world. It's all there for us to discover. Create a blend together based on your combined likes and desires.

"Have you ever lost yourself in a kiss? I mean pure psychedelic inebriation. Not just lustful petting but transcendental metamorphosis when you became aware that the greatness of

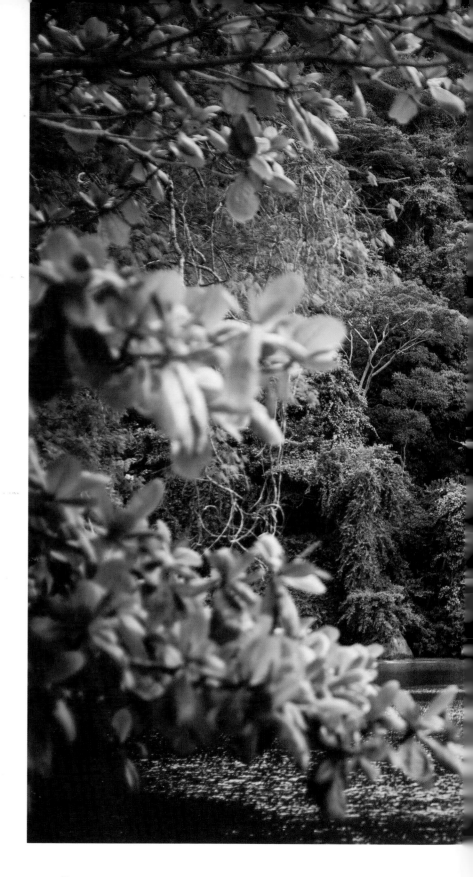

aromatherapy for sensual living *steamy, dreamy, creamy: enthralling essential oil practices*

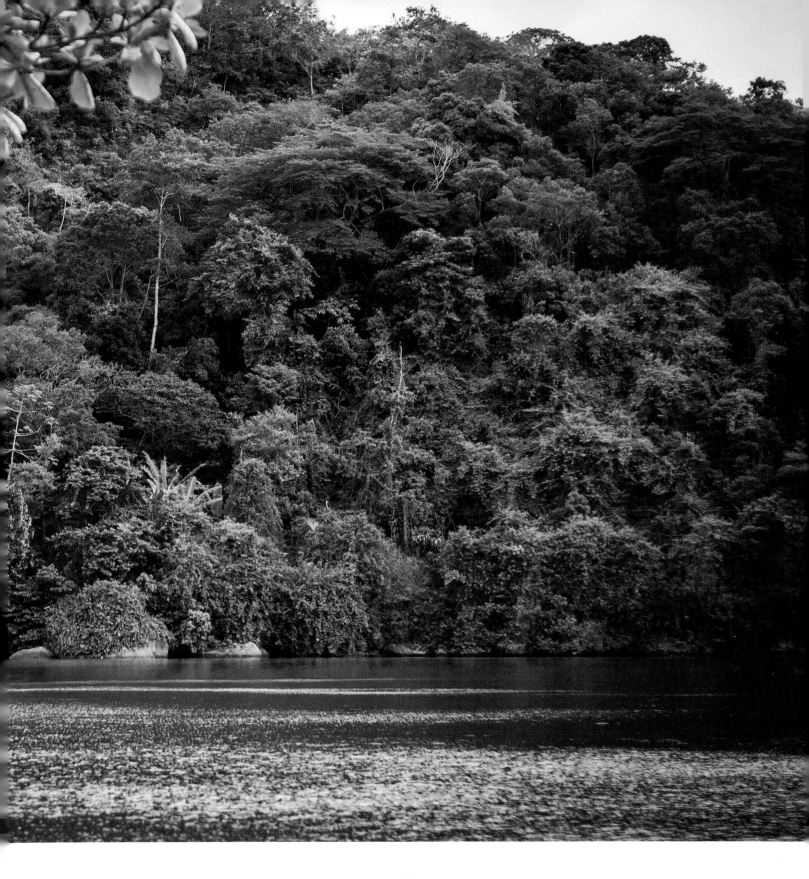

aromatherapy for sensual living   *steamy, dreamy, creamy: enthralling essential oil practices*

this being was breathing into you. Licking the sides and corners of your mouth, like sealing a thousand fleshy envelopes filled with the essence of your passionate being and then opened by the same mouth and delivered back to you, over and over again — the first kiss of the rest of your life. A kiss that confirms that the universe is aligned, that the world's greatest resource is love, and maybe even that God is a woman. With or without a belief in God, all kisses are metaphors decipherable by allocations of time, circumstance, and understanding."

– Saul Williams

Lovely *Lymph Drainage Massage*

Massage and essential oils simply were made for each other. Who doesn't want to be touched, adored, and adorned by their lover with their favorite natural scent? Massage can be amazing if it's done with intention and a little body awareness. I felt it was important to include a simple massage protocol to inform the sensual lover. While oils and massage are made for each other, receiving a bad massage is akin to going to the dentist. You just lie there politely waiting for it to be over without screaming out in pain. A little bit of knowledge goes a long way to help your lover relax, release, recharge, and rev up to be with you in the most intimate of ways.

When I treat someone, I actively tune into his/her body, frequency, and places of stagnation. I step out of the way and allow universal healing energy to flow through my hands to meet the person in whatever he/she needs. I use this invocation at the beginning of every treatment while washing my hands:

"Universal forces of nature, I ask that you come through me while I step aside to serve. I call any and all healing energies that are appropriate for my treatment today with _____. I ask that this treatment is in love, light, and peace, and for the greatest good of all everywhere. Amen. So be it. Aho."

In treatment, I wait patiently with my hands pressed into a congested area while sending loving intentions. I hold for as long as necessary until the body is ready to release. My style of healing is gentle yet deep. I would rather support the flow of energy than fight my way to release congestion. I'm not a pummeler. It's depleting for me and uncomfortable for the client. Feel for the current of energy

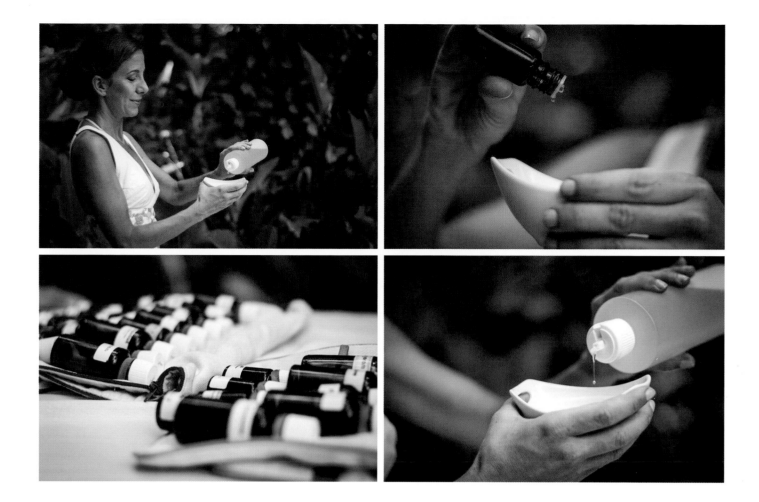

running through your hands and into the person. It's a very powerful currency. As you touch people with intention, valuable information will be revealed as to how long to touch and how much pressure to use.

Let your fingers find spots that are sore, hot, cold, tight, raised, indented, angry, or tired. A congested area can have many different sensations. When it releases, it can feel like a slow, oozing molasses, popping bubble paper, or squeezing a large overdue pimple.

Carrier oils are just as important as pure essential oils in massage. The carrier oils I use are jojoba and coconut oil, as they both have great glide and slide that lasts for a long time. More importantly,

aromatherapy for sensual living *steamy, dreamy, creamy: enthralling essential oil practices*

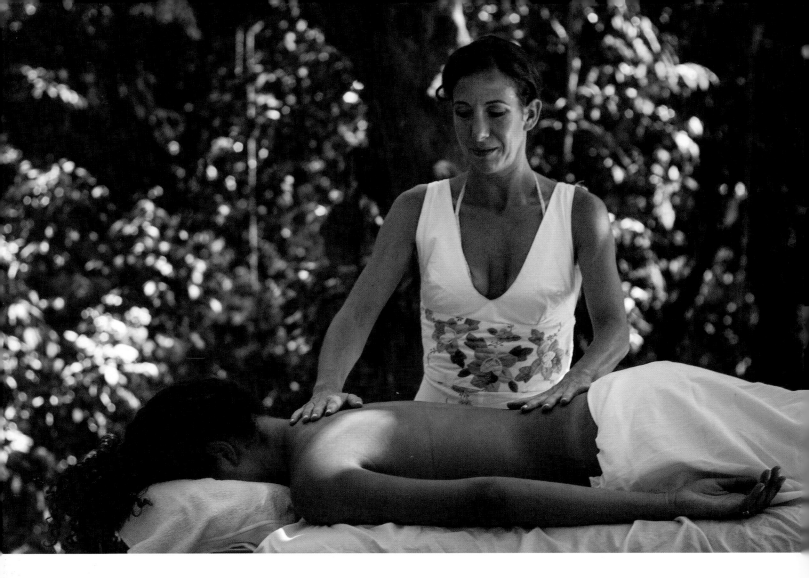

jojoba and coconut oil don't go rancid easily. Carrier oils like sweet almond, apricot, sesame, or even holly oil are often putrid, adulterated, fractionated, or folded — making them potentially toxic to the body.

Blend two tablespoons of your choice of carrier oil and up to a 15 percent dilution of essential oils in a small, shallow bowl. Swirl the essential oils in the carrier oil so they mingle with each other before applying to the skin.

Before you start your massage, take a moment to tune into your lover's body and frequency. Hold a clear intention of what you want your lover to achieve by your massaging him/her. You have an enormous ability to infuse the massage with spine-tingling sexiness or the earnest desire to heal and hold

aromatherapy for sensual living   *steamy, dreamy, creamy: enthralling essential oil practices*

the one you love. Touch is powerful, even transcendent. Your thoughts plus the addition of powerful essential oils will greatly impact the nature of the session. Choose wisely.

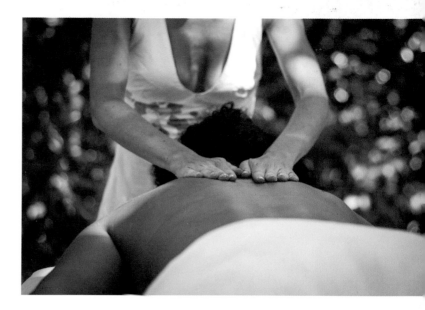

- Have your lover lie on his/her stomach and cover the lower body with a sheet and a blanket. Being warm and cozy is essential to a good massage. Place a small amount of oil in your hands and take a moment to allow it to warm up before touching the body. Your body heat, intention, and unique personal energy will infuse into the medicinal and aromatic properties of the oils to help your lover relax and receive.

- Ask your lover to take three deep and long breaths. At the beginning of the third exhalation, meet his/her breath with your touch. Feel free to time your breath to theirs.

- Start at the tops of the shoulders and sweep down the spine to the sacrum with both hands. Sweep or effleurage back up to the shoulders to cover the whole back with oil. Make large, steady, slow ovals with deliberate hands. Effleurage at least five times. Kindly avoid pressing directly on the spine or any joint. That never feels good. Also remember to touch the body with all ten of your fingers. Sometimes thumbs or pinkies stick up and make the treatment feel awkward or incomplete. Check with your partner to see if

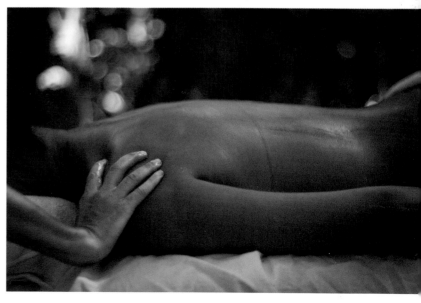

aromatherapy for sensual living *steamy, dreamy, creamy: enthralling essential oil practices*

he/she wants more or less pressure. Knowing purrs are a good indication that you're doing it right.

- When you've covered the entire back with oil, use both hands to feel into the shoulders and neck with small circular movements. Release feels utterly sublime, especially when met by loving aromatic hands. With firm but moderate pressure, make small and precise circles with your thumbs, fingers, and/or heels of your hands to gently loosen and release any tightness you encounter. Some tender spots to look out for are underneath the shoulder blade, at the base of the neck, at the sides of the neck, at the occipital ridge (where the hair meets the neck), and one inch down from where the neck meets the shoulders.

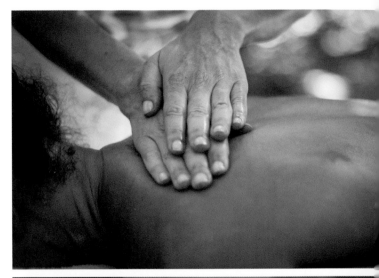

- Place yourself on the left side of the body. Gently milk the neck by pulling the flesh up with alternate hands to release tension and stress. Make sure that you go over the entire length of the neck and then move to the right side of the body to ensure that the neck receives the strength of both thumbs.

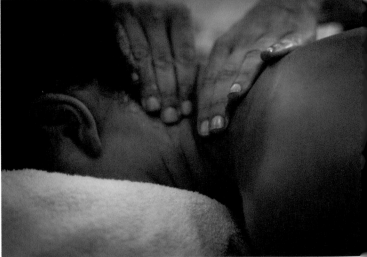

- Stand again at the left shoulder with your body perpendicular to theirs. Place one hand on top of the other and slide a full open palm across the left shoulder blade, working toward the middle line. Move down and across the skinny part

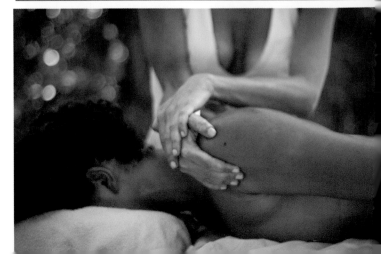

of the blade and then up the side of the body. You're making a triangle over the shoulder blades with your hands. Do this several times with firm pressure on both sides to complete the shoulder region.

- Cup the left shoulder with one hand on top of the other. Gently pull the shoulder up and back with alternate hands at the joint to release shoulder tightness. This move is particularly effective with those who hunch their shoulders or have trouble opening their hearts. With gentle force, imagine that you're helping them to spread their wings.

- Go back to the tension-filled parts of the shoulders and neck to spend additional time releasing those areas. Use the pressure from your thumb on the knobby parts, kneading back and forth, to release.

- Move over to the right side of the body and do the same movements.

- Move to the lower back. On the left side, cover the area with oil from the sacrum (the bony protrusion at the bottom part of the spine) to the top of the shoulder in an effleurage motion.

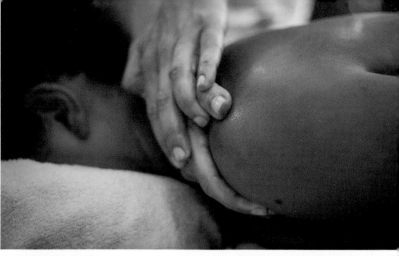

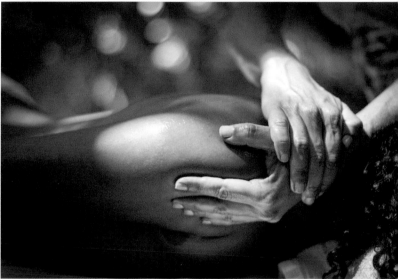

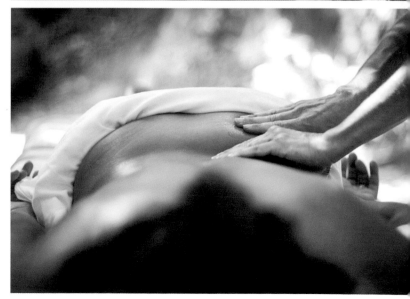

- At the base of the sacrum, spread fingers wide apart. Follow one hand behind the other from the left sacrum up to the left shoulder, and then chase down the side of the body as though the hands are trailing each other.

- Rearrange the sheets to uncover the sacrum, gluteals, and hips while being mindful to cover the sensitive bits and pieces. Lovingly anoint the entire area with oil and deeply massage. It might start to get a little hot. Try your best to simmer down.

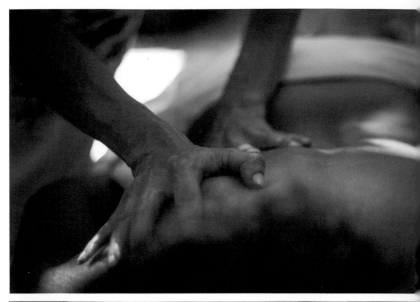

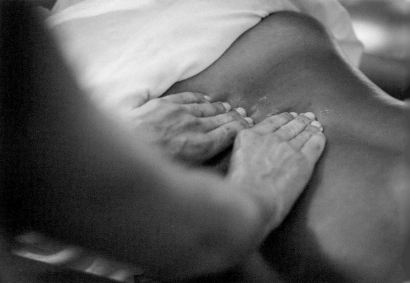

- Rest both hands on the sacrum on either side of the spine. With your thumbs, feel for the quarter-sized nodules or divots where the sciatic nerves come out of the spine. This can be a very sensitive spot for many. Slowly massage the nodules in small circles with your thumb (while your fingers spread out in a fan over the sacrum). Check with your partner to see if the pressure is sufficient.

- Gently milk and massage the cheeks with both hands in a rhythmic fashion. It's a big muscle so take time to do a thorough job.

- Place your elbow in the center of the gluteal muscle with medium pressure and then allow it to slide out to the side of the body. Do this with moderate care, as it can be tender for

aromatherapy for sensual living *steamy, dreamy, creamy: enthralling essential oil practices*

those with a (ahem) tight ass. There's nothing finer than receiving a deep gluteal massage. It's quite sexy, too.

- Complete this section by moving over to the right side and doing the same movements on the other side of the body. At this point, you've covered the neck, shoulders, back, and gluteal muscles. Do an effleurage sweep up on the whole back and then cover it with a sheet or towel to complete.

- Move down to the legs. Uncover the right leg and saturate it with oil using the same effleurage motion that you did on the back.

- With your back facing your partner's head, sweep up the inner leg with one hand following the other all the way up, using moderate pressure and avoiding the back of the knee. This will help lymphatic flow and touch some really sensitive tissue. Keep it clean here. It's not the time to explore the heavenly gate.

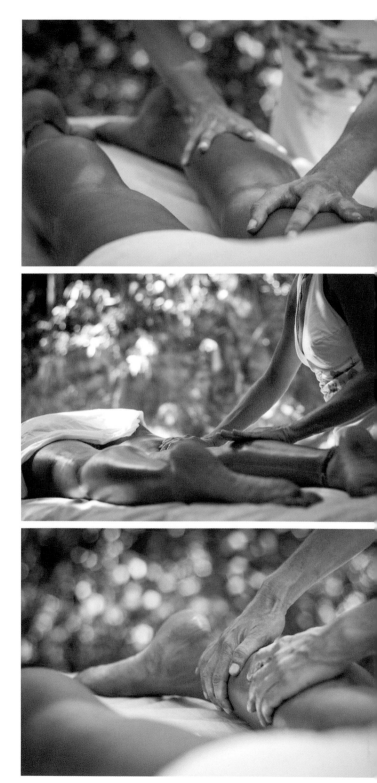

aromatherapy for sensual living *steamy, dreamy, creamy: enthralling essential oil practices*

- Lift the foot up so the leg is in an L shape with the foot in the air and thigh facing down. Milk the area behind the ankle with the thumb and forefinger (while using the other hand to support the foot).

- While still supporting the foot, use the heel of your hand to move down the center of the calf, moving out to the lateral and then back up to meet the ankle. Do this several times. Gently return the leg to the bed with grace, being careful not to squish the toes.

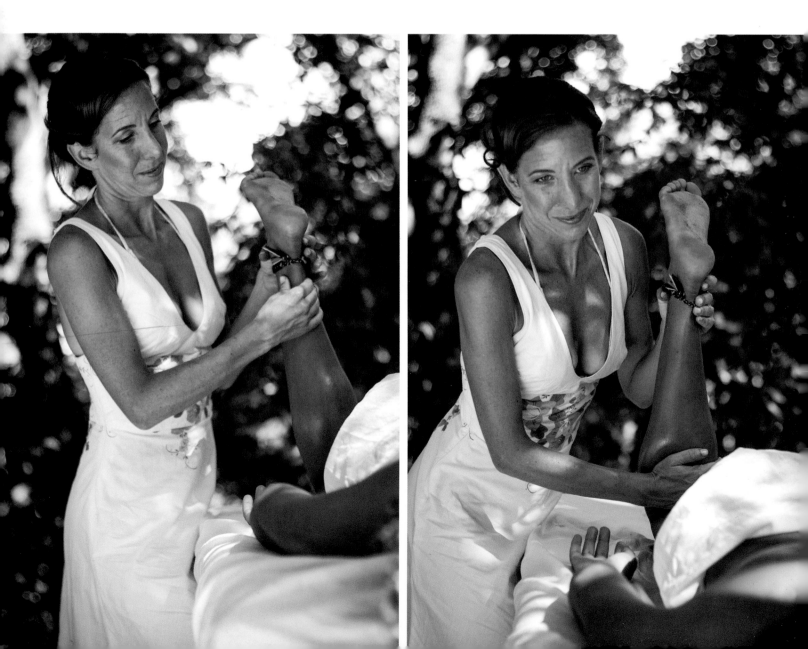

- Stand at their feet. With both thumbs on one leg, start at the back of the ankle and glide up the middle to split the calf and then go around and back down to the ankle. It's as though you're drawing the seam of a stocking on their leg. Complete this movement three times.

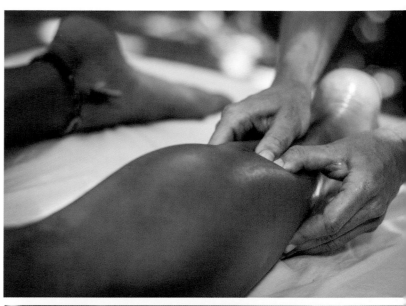

- Standing at the hip, guide the legs open slightly. Using the full palm and fingers, gently sweep up the interior flesh of the leg to the high inner thigh. Complete this movement slowly and with strong intent. It will drive your lover crazy with desire.

- Starting at the ankle, trace the index finger and thumb up the back of the leg to land at the base of the gluteal (where the hip meets the bottom). Press firmly

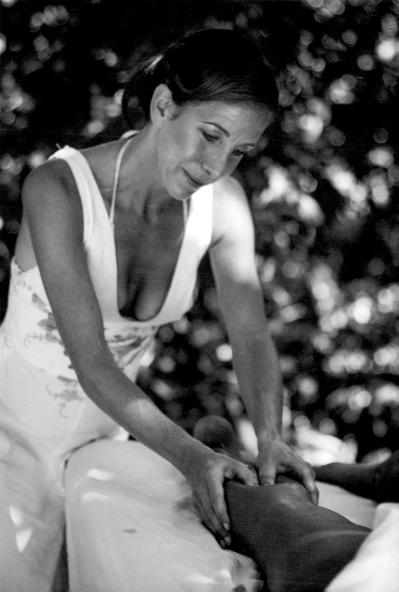

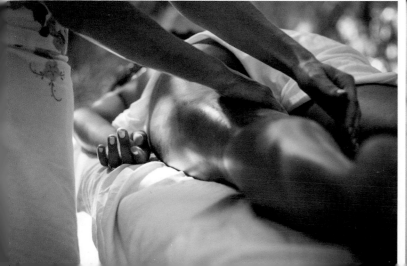

for fifteen to thirty seconds in the nodule. The area should feel congested and, when pressed, you should feel a release of energy. Trace the fingers for a second time up to the outer nodule at the center of the piriformis muscle. Press firmly for fifteen to thirty seconds. You'll feel a release.

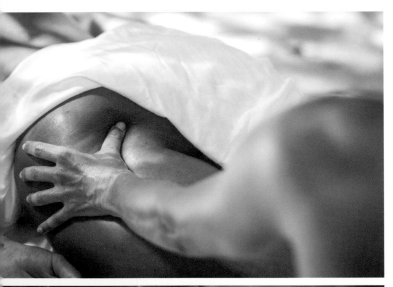

- Standing at the ankle with your back toward your partner's head, sweep up the leg with one hand over the other all the way up the leg, again avoiding the back of the knee. Do this a few times, always moving toward the heart (never down). Move on to the right leg to repeat the entire sequence.

- You've now completed the entire back of the body. Place your hands on your partner's back for a moment and then ask him/her to slowly turn over on to the back. Readjust the sheets so the person is covered and comfortable. Now is a good time to steal a kiss.

- While still at the legs, cover the front of the right leg with oil in the effleurage motion.

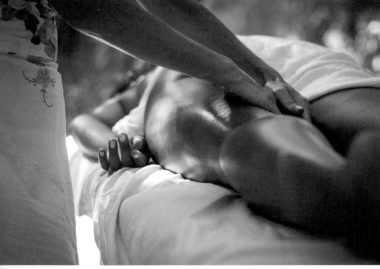

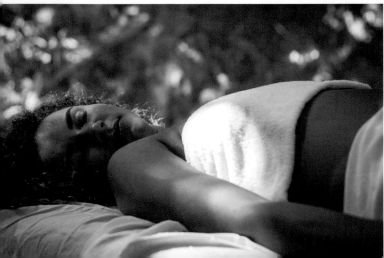

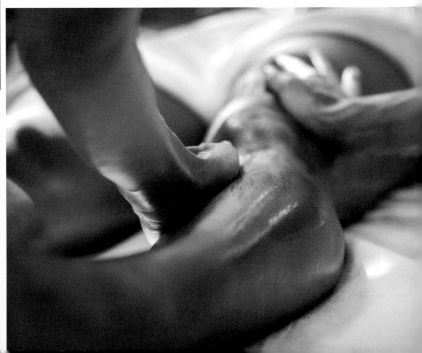

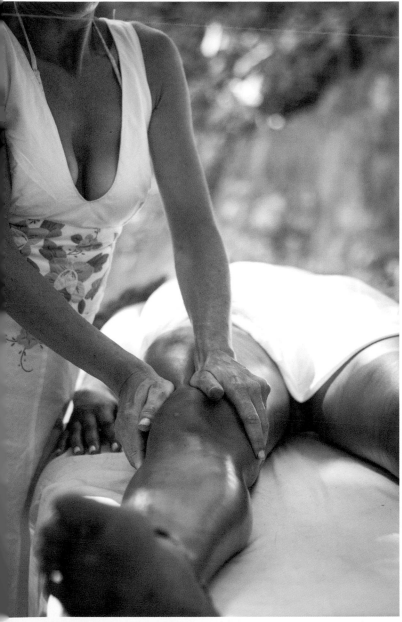

- Move so your back is toward your partner's head. Gently pull the skin up from the inner ankle to the inner thigh with alternating hands. Use firm pressure. Be sure to cover the entire surface while staying toward the midline of the body.

- Place one hand above the knee. With the other hand, straddle the shin with the thumb and fingers resting at the base of the ankle. Gently yet firmly glide up the shin to the knee to remove any stagnant goo stored in the shin muscle. Do this three times. It feels like you're pushing toothpaste out of a tube.

- With hands above the knee, at the lowest part of the thigh, and fingers pointing to the toes, milk down the flesh on either side of the knee to disperse accumulation in the knee joint. Milk three times. Please don't place direct pressure on the knee.

- Keeping one hand above the knee, move the other hand below the knee and turn fingers toward each other. Using the thumb and fingers, allow one hand to gently squeeze and massage the flesh in an alternate rhythm.

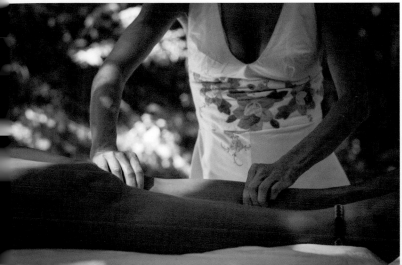

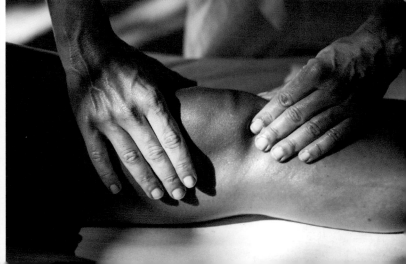

- Turn your body toward the head of your lover. Smile mischievously. Use the heel of your hand. With firm pressure, move from just above the knee up the centerline of the thigh, and massage around the hip bone and down the side. Do this several times, as many people hold tension in their legs. It will be a welcome release.

- Move to the feet and lightly pull the leg from the socket to release tension. Now is also a great time to give a foot massage. Love is in the details.

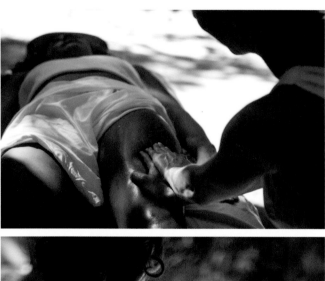

- Rotate the ankles, gently pull the toes, and massage the entire foot from top to bottom. The longer you spend the on the feet, the happier your love friend will be.

- Complete the whole massage sequence on the other leg. Cover the legs with sheets.

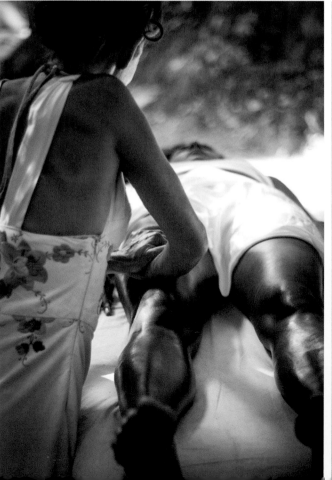

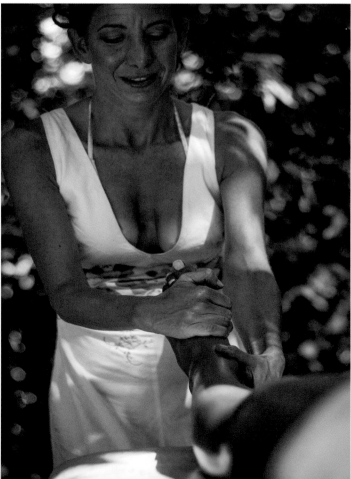

- Move to the stomach, revealing the chest if appropriate (and warm), otherwise cover the chest with a small towel and pull down the sheet to the pubic line. Apply oil all over the stomach in a clockwise motion. For many people, it feels really good to massage deeply into the pockets of the abdomen and to knead the skin. You'll help digestion, detoxify major organs, and treat an area that rarely gets touched.

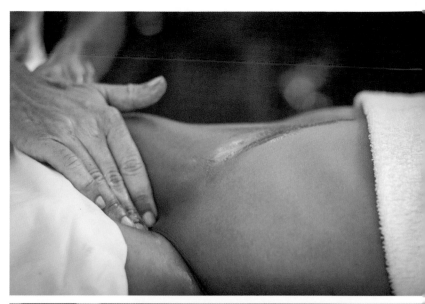

- Cover the whole stomach in a clockwise rotation for at least three rotations.

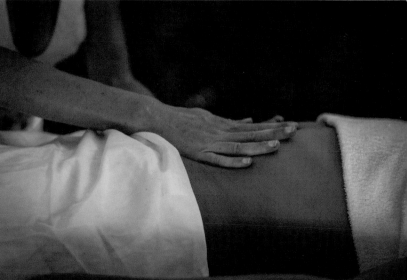

- Move to the solar plexus (halfway between the belly button and the sternum). Gently massage the area with one hand on top of the other in small counter-clockwise circles. This can be sensitive for some, especially those who suffer from a great deal of stress. Visualize the color yellow and send calm and loving energy.

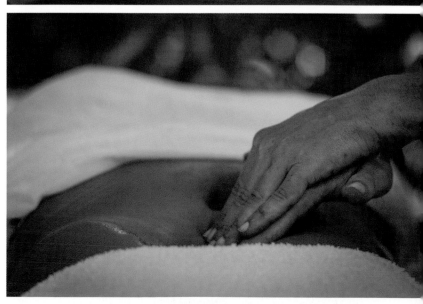

- Move to the chakra point below the navel (the sacral plexus) and gently work in small clockwise circles. You'll quite often feel an energetic pull to the correct spot. Hold your original intention for the massage. Your partner will feel it through his/her sexual center. Sometimes

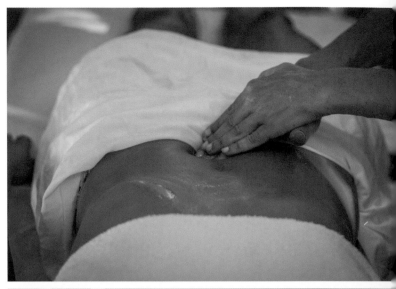

thoughts, visions, words, or experiences can come to you while resting in this spot. Remember to tell your lover later. Please be aware that this can be a sensitive spot for some, especially if there's been sexual trauma or surgery.

- With your hands on either side of the body, gently pull up on the fleshy parts on the sides of the abdomen to release the kidneys and adrenals. Pull up and hold for five to ten seconds, twice.

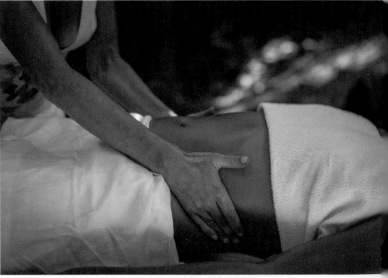

- Complete the stomach by massaging in clockwise circles using both hands all over the stomach. Cover the stomach and chest with the sheet.

- Gently uncover the arms from the sheet. On the right, apply oil to the arm in the effleurage motion, using both hands one after the other to cover the entire arm on both sides.

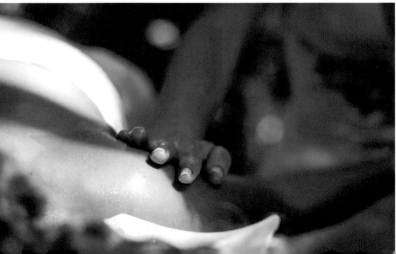

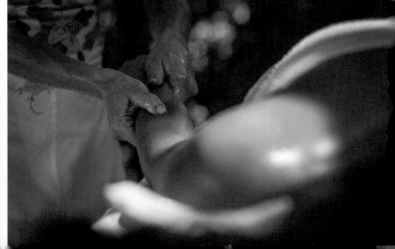

- Hold the arm in one hand. With the other hand, use the thumb to firmly go up the center of the forearm, starting from back of the hand and sweeping down around the sides. Massage into the muscle three times with both thumbs to cover different muscles in the forearm. Flip the arm over to do the interior aspect of the forearm with the same motions.

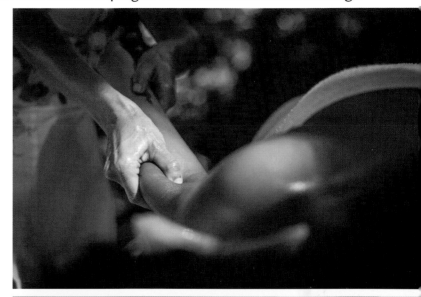

- Move down to the hands. Gently wiggle and pull each finger. Deeply massage the fleshy pad below the thumbs and squeeze the pad between the thumb and forefinger.

- Interlace your fingers in theirs. Give the wrist a full rotation in both directions three times each. Allow a slow unwinding, as it heightens intimacy. On the top of the hand, use your thumb and forefinger to press down into the fleshy parts between each finger and then move down toward the wrist.

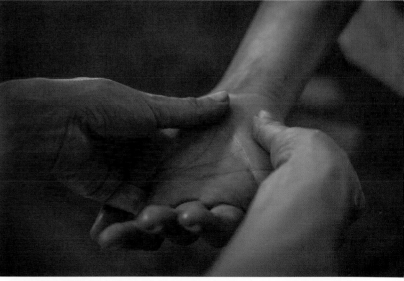

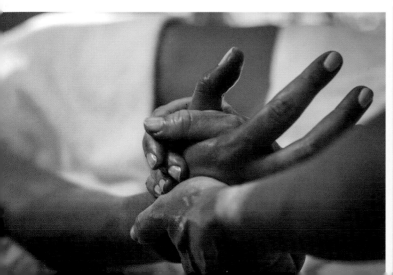

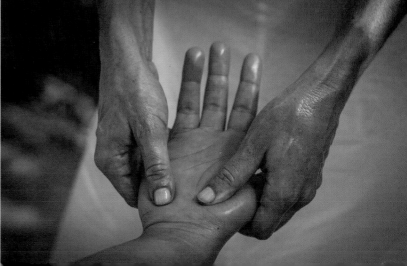

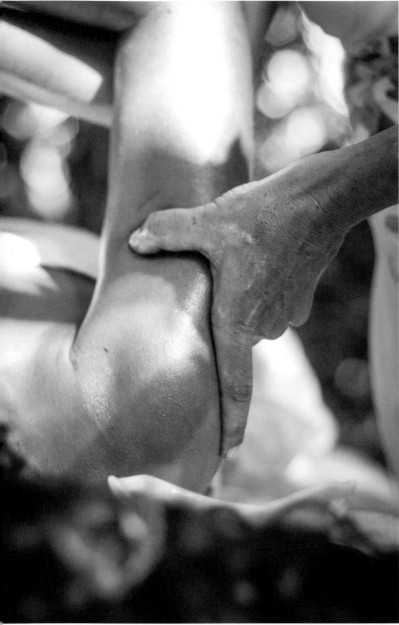

- Place the arm in an L shape with the hand above the heart. With your other hand, knead and massage the bicep, triceps, and interior aspect of the upper arm. Do this at least three times for each muscle.

- Massage the entire arm from wrist to shoulder with alternating hands in an effleurage motion to complete.

- Perform the same motions on the left arm. Place both arms back underneath the sheet.

- Move up to the head. Place a small amount of oil on the face. The great news is that pure essential oils and carrier oils don't cause acne breakouts. In fact, they do a lot to regenerate skin, improve elasticity, and reduce wrinkles, puffiness, and red spots.

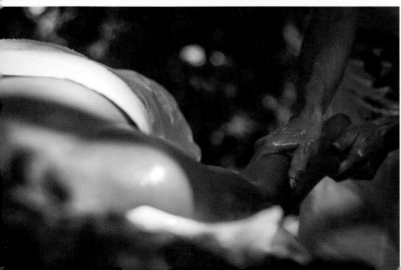

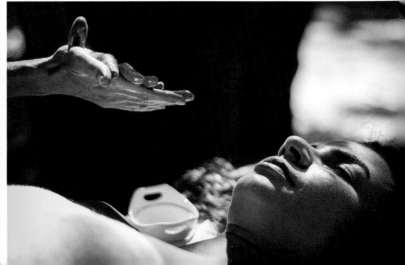

- With your fingertips, gently massage down from the forehead to the cheeks to the chin, and sweep out to the ears.

- Gently pull the ears, starting at the lobe and moving to the top. There are many nerve endings in the ears that just love to be touched and adored. Do this a few times. Resist the urge to nibble and suck on the lobes.

- Move to the jaw line and rest your fingers between the two biting surfaces on the cheeks. Slowly massage in circular movements and exert a small amount of pressure to the area to release a tight jaw. The masseter is the strongest muscle in the body and often the tightest. By releasing it through massage and essential oils, you'll help your lover sail effortlessly into blissful rapture. This is also a move you can do on yourself to release stress and tension.

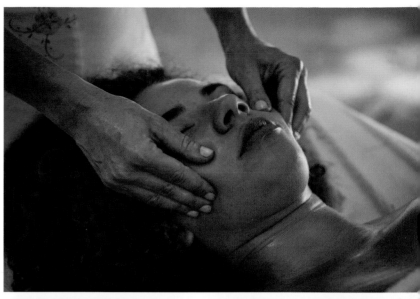

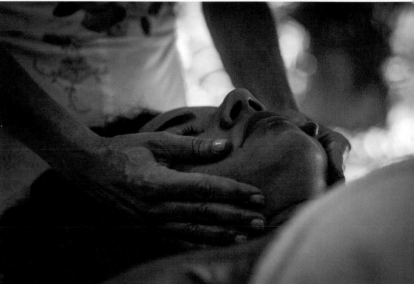

- Support the head as you slowly turn it to the side. With the non-supporting hand, use your fingertips to massage deeply into the side neck muscles from the base of the skull down to the clavicle. Do this at least three times on either side.

- Rest your hands on the top of the head. Allow yourself some time to tune into your partner's frequency and help him/her relax deeper. This is a critical moment in the massage. Take at least two to five minutes to feel any sensations, tingling, or magnetic pulls on the scalp. It's a sacred time. Your lover will appreciate the attention you have given to him/her and probably reward you with a massage of your own.

- Finish the massage by gently pressing your thumbs into the arches of the feet. Hold for at least one minute. Send a silent prayer to your lover. Send peace, good wishes and vibrant health. If it's appropriate, slip in something slightly taboo.

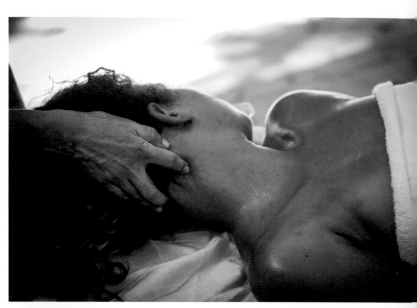

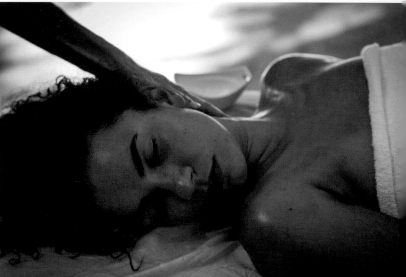

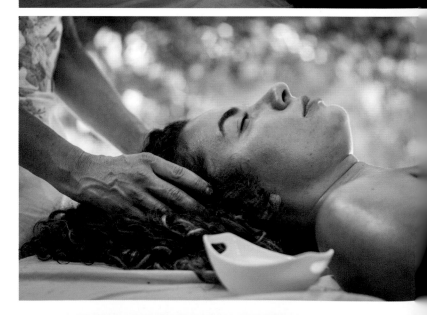

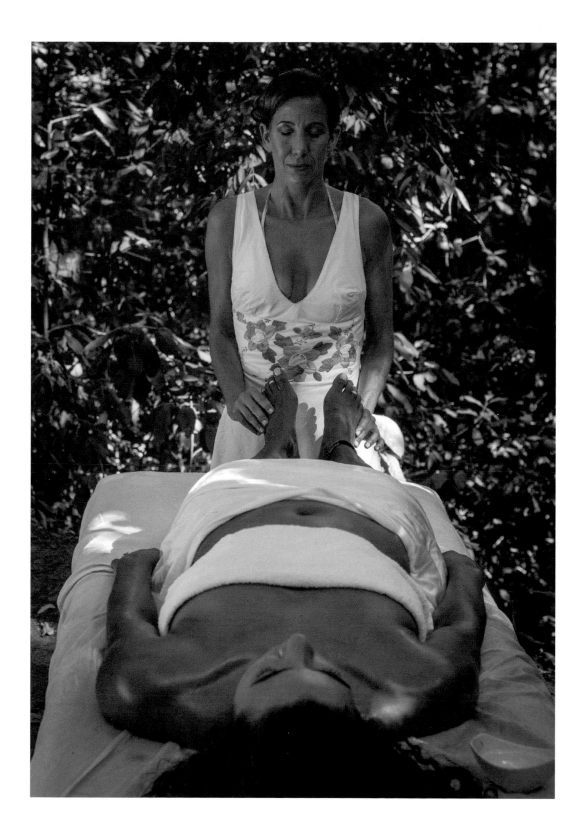

aromatherapy for sensual living *steamy, dreamy, creamy: enthralling essential oil practices*

Some salacious massage oil combinations are:

- Cardamom, sandalwood, black pepper
- Ylang ylang, lemon, cinnamon
- Cape chamomile, immortelle, lavender
- Jasmine, tangerine, vanilla
- Ginger, grapefruit, vanilla
- Cacao, vanilla, black pepper
- Neroli, lavender, sandalwood
- Cinnamon, tangerine, vanilla
- Tuberose, lavender, lemon
- Sandalwood, geranium, ginger
- Fenugreek, vanilla, black pepper

Stimulating *Breast Massage*

Women's breasts are the embodiment of femininity. They provide sustenance for babes and are symbols of beauty. Sadly, our breasts have been stuffed, pushed up, grabbed, and are feared as the carriers of disease. Many women don't yet practice regular health-fortifying breast massage and often their partners overlook or don't know the importance of breast play in sexual exchange. It makes for some very sad ta-tas. Sex can be so much more stimulating for women with dedicated time for breast massage. Interestingly, the breasts are a direct line into a woman's two main pleasure centers — her brain and vagina — and situated conveniently at her heart center.

aromatherapy for sensual living *steamy, dreamy, creamy: enthralling essential oil practices*

By massaging the breasts, you'll help to firm them, boost the flow of the lymphatic immune system, and help to excrete excess estrogen, thus improving breast and hormonal health. Using essential oils and carriers in breast massage will only heighten the experience for both you and your lover.

The breasts extend from the underarm to the sixth rib and to the center of the chest. Be sure to incorporate all skin and tissue to have a full and complete massage.

This massage can be done solo or with a partner and can even be done on men. It can be a welcomed surprise and a way to treat their sensitive and sometimes guarded hearts.

- Start with one tablespoon of coconut or olive oil and up to three erotic, edible essential oils. Warm the oil in your hands for two minutes and then pour just enough in your hands to cover both breasts. Spread the oil over the breasts, going from the center line in the middle of the chest toward the underarm area and down in large circular movements.

- Caress the breasts slowly and gently. Using the entire palm of your hand over the whole breast, palpating to activate the massage. Try to create a rhythm so your partner can time his/her breathing to your touch.

- Place your hands over the breast with the nipple in the center of your palm. Spread your fingers to cover the whole breast like spokes of a wheel. Pull the fingers away from the breast so the fingertips land on the nipples. Go back and forth with this motion. Finish off with a gentle pinch.

- Gently massage each breast by lifting it up and pressing softly like you would knead bread. The undersides of breasts are particularly sensitive and most women enjoy a soft touch in this area. The flesh can also be twisted and wrung very gently.

- Using just your fingertips, stroke the full breast with clockwise and then counterclockwise caresses.

Now you can move to directly massaging the nipples.

- Place both thumbs on one breast and place them on opposite sides of her nipple, starting at the outside edge of her areola. Slowly and gently bring your thumbs together, lightly squeezing her nipple between your thumbs, and pull outward toward you. Repeat this until you make a complete circle around her nipples.

- Be sure to adjust the pressure depending on how she reacts. Some women like it hard while some prefer a softer touch.

- Gently massage the breast in circular movements, going from the center out toward the sides. Repeat the whole sequence on the other breast.

Using your mouth, tongue, and teeth is also a very effective way to stimulate. Pretend that you're slowly eating a succulent and juicy mango. You can slowly kiss and suck her nipples. Use your tongue in circular motions around the areola while gently cupping her breasts with your hand. A gentle, well-timed blow on the breasts can blow her mind. You can use your teeth to graze and nibble, but never bite.

Essential oils on the breasts are riveting for a woman. Some — like cinnamon, clove, black pepper, ginger, and cardamom — are mildly warming and will bring blood and energy to the breasts. With warming oils, use only one drop as they can be sensitive to some and cause mild irritation. Oils like rose otto and geranium will intensify the feelings of admiration and affection between lovers. Oils like ylang ylang, immortelle, vanilla, and sandalwood are pure aphrodisiacs and will heighten any sexual encounter. They taste delicious, too.

Some combinations of erotic oils to use on the breasts are:

- Clove and rose otto
- Cinnamon and lemon
- Tangerine and immortelle
- Cape chamomile and vanilla
- Lemon and sandalwood
- Ginger and grapefruit

- Cardamom and vanilla

- Rose otto and lavender (This is deeply healing to those who've experienced sexual violence or heartbreak.)

- Bergamot and ylang ylang

- Cape chamomile and immortelle

Aromatic *Kissing*

Oh the delights of the lips . . . kissing is so telling of the warmth and connection between lovers. The lips are one of the most sensitive parts of the body, with dense sense receptors that respond so well to loving touch. Kissing is even more delightful when combined with the perfect power of pure perfume.

Drop one essential oil on a teaspoon of raw honey. Take turns feeding the combination to each other, slowly, methodically, and with dimmed lights. Slowly meet your lover's lips. Gently blow the aromatic nectar between your mouths. Taste the honeyed bliss and ascend. Another option is to select two complementary oils such as rose otto and vanilla; ylang ylang and lemon; or frankincense and fenugreek. Place an individual oil on two small pieces of chocolate. Bring your lips together to smooch. Allow the essential oils to mix and mingle in your mouths, creating a liquid light of sensual bliss.

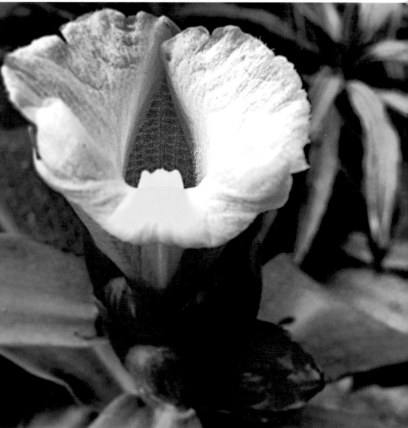

aromatherapy for sensual living *steamy, dreamy, creamy: enthralling essential oil practices*

Petal *Power*

The deepest and most sensuous way I know how to use essential oils is applying them on the petals of a woman. This is an astoundingly seductive practice that will completely blow your lover's mind. It also feels really good on you too. Because of the antifungal, antiviral, antibiotic nature of essential oils, they'll also help to treat female reproductive disorders like candida, bacterial vaginosis, vaginal dryness, or general itchiness. Using essential oils in the most intimate places will also cause your skin to plump in the most marvelous way.

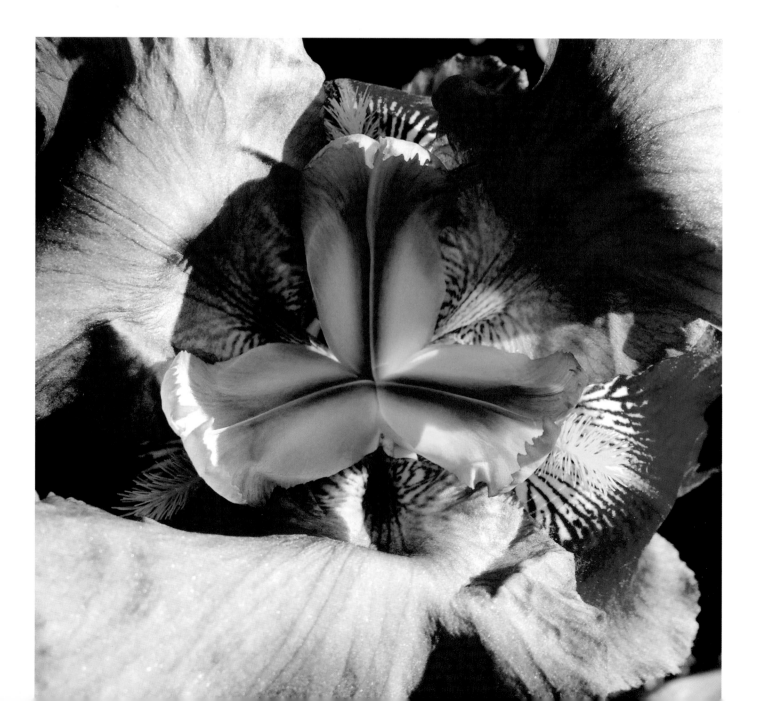

You can adorn your petals before a big date or just before you start to make love. Remember to smooth oils down to your inner thighs as well. I adore having an aromatic surprise for my lovers and for myself. The oils commingle with your personal scent to create a fragrance that's completely and deliciously unique to you. Your lover also receives all the euphoric, aphrodisiac, high-making properties of the oils when he intimately greets you. That is a win-win.

Vaginal skin is considerably thinner and more porous than dermis in other parts of the body. It's therefore even more important to only use natural lubrication products for lovemaking. Essential oils are potent. For petal adornment, only use one drop of oil in one tablespoon of coconut oil, shea butter, and jojoba and/or cacao cream. Your desire is to flavor the petals rather than overpower. (However, if you're using essential oils to treat a specific vaginal condition, blend in higher concentrations.) One tablespoon goes a long way. Keep it stored in an airtight container or use it all in one session as an all-over love lube.

Petal adornment is a fantastic way to treat and heal delicate tissue after an intense, rambunctious roll in the hay. It will soothe soft and supple skin so there is less pain, itchiness, or rawness. Urinate and wash with non-toxic soap after sex and adorn those petals slowly and lovingly. It's a deep act of self-love and nurturance. It's also fun to let him adorn you.

There are many safe and healing oils that are wonderfully appropriate for your petals. You can also make a combination of these oils to customize a personal love lube.

Some petal-adornment oils are rosewood, geranium, cape chamomile, sandalwood, lavender, neroli, ylang ylang, vanilla, rose otto, cardamom, immortelle, and fenugreek.

Glistening

Glistening is the practice of adorning yourself in public (or private) whenever there's an unpleasant aroma emanating from you or your environment. When I'm in the subway or at a sweaty dance party, I always have a bottle of something euphoric or exotic (or a combination) to adorn myself. A lady never leaves home without aromatic enhancements. This practice helps to continuously boost my immune system, and I love that I leave an aromatic impression wherever I go.

We are attracted to people who have a pleasant personal aroma; it's an innate understanding of one's health and vitality. I invite you to explore glistening whenever you encounter a bad smell. People will definitely take notice as smell is undeniable.

To *My Pregnant Sisters*

Many books scare women into believing that essential oils are a gigantic pregnancy no-no. I disagree. Essential oils brilliantly harmonize with every aspect of a woman's life and reproductive cycle, and can be deeply curative throughout pregnancy.

There are some recommendations to follow, such as only using medicinal-grade, authentic essential oils from reputable companies (like www.purfrequency.com). Many oils found in the health food store or through MLM companies are less than pure and can be downright toxic; limit internal applications to one single drop a day and generously dilute in water, juice, olive oil or in a smoothie; in massage, apply essential oils in a maximum 2–5 percent dilution (less is more because of pregnant women's sensitivity to smell); and use them consciously and in moderation.

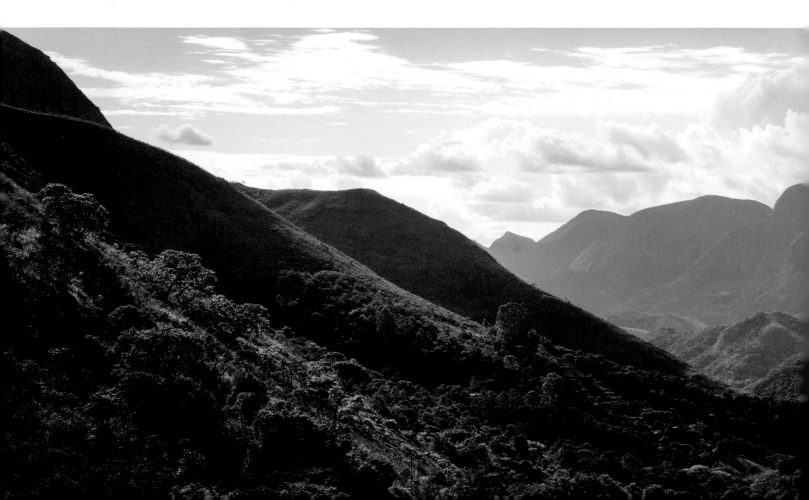

I invite you to trust your womanly intuition when using essential oils at this time.

Some oils that should be avoided in pregnancy include:

- Fennel: can be an abortifacient and bring in breast milk too early.

- Sage: can cause milk to dry up.

- Jasmine: can induce premature labor, though this is unlikely.

- Cinnamon: can cause blood to circulate too quickly.

- Clove: can overwhelm a pregnant woman.

- Wintergreen: can be too stimulating for you and the baby. (This is an oil that shouldn't be used.)

Be mindful, mama, but don't give into fear and let that stop you from using other essential oils. Endlessly generous, they will help to inform and empower this sacred moment in your life. I would rather use a drop of essential oil to balance the body than pop potentially health-suppressing drugs. Always be responsible with the amount you are using and there shouldn't be any adverse reactions. Essential oils are most helpful in the second and third trimester.

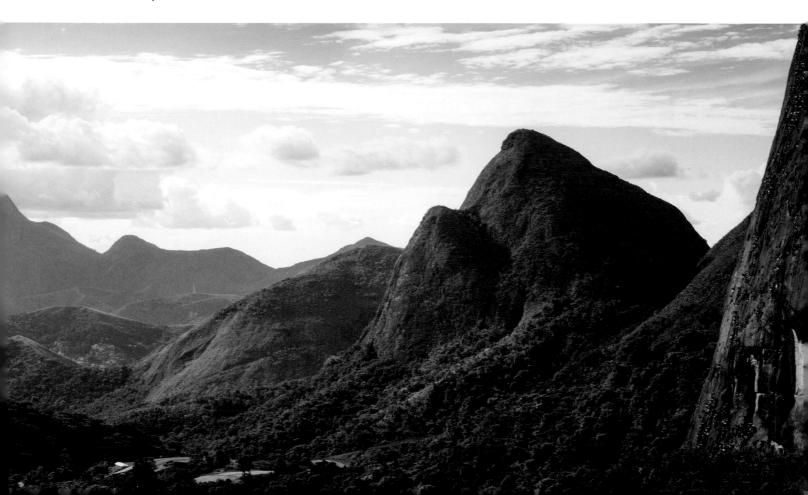

There is infinite intelligence in the plants to help you harmonize with the new life you are nurturing, soothe any aches, pains, or anxieties, and make you feel brilliantly, gorgeously awesome. Love is in the flowers.

In the birthing process, trust your body's ingrained biological knowledge. It is wise. Invite a maximum level of surrender in every divine breath. Let the essential oils be the bridge to help you get to the blissful birthing place. Keep connecting with your little babe's spirit to help him/her feel at ease in making their transition. Relax and surrender.

Some splendid, enlivening oils to use in pregnancy are:

- Neroli
- Tangerine
- Cape chamomile
- Cardamom
- Grapefruit
- Petitgrain
- Ginger (excellent for nausea)
- Lavender
- Frankincense

- Peppermint (small amounts)
- Patchouli
- Ylang ylang
- Juniper
- Eucalyptus
- Bergamot
- Cypress
- Tea tree oil
- Geranium

Methods *of Use*

One or two methods a day is more than sufficient during pregnancy. Less is more.

Baths are an excellent way to receive essential oils. For pregnancy, use four or five drops. One of the simplest baths is lavender with one tablespoon of coconut oil. Foot baths with one to two drops (especially in the third trimester) can be a wonderful healing and relaxing experience.

Diffuse a mild aromatic blend while sleeping. It's good for you and the baby. Use only four or five drops in the diffuser. Continue to use the same blend once the baby is born so he/she too can relax and surrender to the flowers.

During labor, use lavender on the back, third eye, and/or between the pinkie and ring finger on wrist to tone the heart points. It will relieve tension and emotional stress during the process of labor.

My favorite and most effective birthing blend is jasmine, lavender, marjoram, petitgrain, and frankincense. Make a 10 percent blend in jojoba and apply it with warm compresses or massage to the low back and pelvic region. It will make contractions stronger and labor shorter. I first made this blend for a pregnant client in Japan. It was so successful that it was distributed to a slew of her pregnant friends, resulting in happy, healthy deliveries.

To help milk come in, use fennel and fenugreek diluted in coconut, jojoba, or olive oil and massage into breasts.

To stop milk flow, use sage diluted in coconut, jojoba, or olive oil and massage into breasts.

Deepening *Sensuality: Pick Up the Perfume of Plants*

Essential oils are everywhere for us to use. This is an excellent exercise to get you physically more in touch with nature and provide you with on the spot aromatherapy when in need. Many of us have a subtle disconnection from or, worse, fear of the natural world. Nature is here for us to share, use, explore, and heal.

Touch plants, feel flowers, and love leaves. They're aching for your caress. Observe the softness of the petals on your skin. It might just be the softest thing in the world and is endlessly exciting to eager fingertips.

To anoint yourself with on the spot aromatherapy, simply rub both hands on any aromatic plant, cover your mouth and nose with your hands, and then inhale deeply. Take a moment to feel the medicinal and aromatic compounds enter your body. If you have a bug bite or difficulty breathing, most aromatic garden plants will help with this method. There is medicine everywhere.

Some aromatic plants to use for this method are lavender, sage, pine needles, jasmine, tuberose, orange skin, rosemary, thyme, parsley, tarragon, marjoram, oregano, geranium, basil, peppermint, and roses.

How *to Make Floral Waters*

Floral waters are simply heavenly and surprisingly easy to make. Floral waters (different than hydrosols) are excellent for imparting aromatic and medicinal properties directly into cells, boosting skin's radiance, and helping to ease a broken heart. Pick a couple of handfuls of flowers (organic is best), place them in a sterilized mason jar, and cover them with fresh spring water. Place the covered jar in the sun for six to twelve hours to allow the sun to infuse the water with floral medicines. Once complete, strain the flowers out. Store the floral water in a cool and dark place for up to six months.

Another option is placing the jar in the moonlight to immerse the floral waters with the potent, watery, and womanly energy of the moon.

Spray floral waters on your face, use as a douche, or drink it in full concentration or in a homeopathic dilution. Flower waters are light in their aromatic composition but very effective in their medicinal aspects. They are wonderful additions to food which impart a witchy, magical, aromatic effect to your plate.

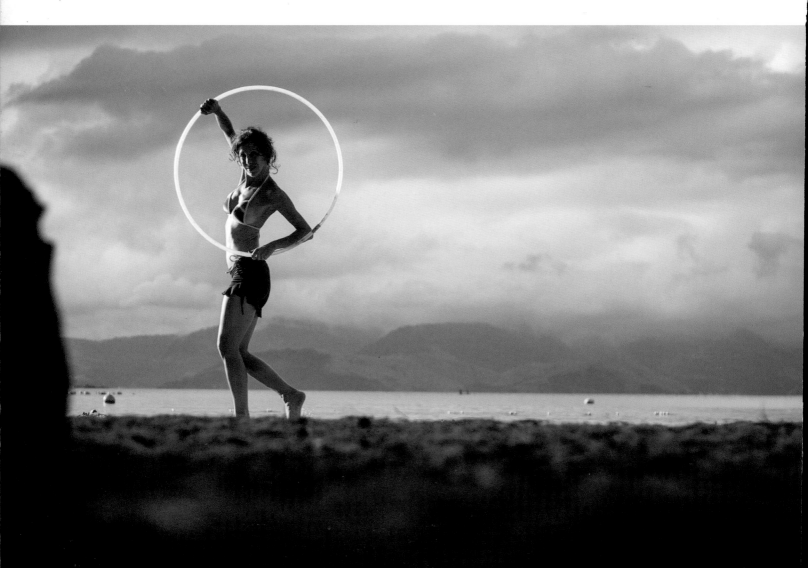

Infusions

Infusing oils with herbs is an excellent witchy way to augment the flavor of your cooking oils and impart medicinal and aromatic properties. Place herbs, garlic, essential oils, aromatic flowers, and/or chilies in a clean and sealable bottle. Cover the plant material with organic olive oil. Allow the plants to infuse with the oils for at least a month. Turn over the bottles every day to invigorate the infusion and equally disperse the medicine. Use the infused oil in salad dressings, stir-fries, eggs, or anywhere you want to impart a strong flavor to your food. Infused oil will keep for up to six months. Once the oil has been infused, please store in the refrigerator.

Vinegars

Use the same method for vinegars as you would for infusion. The best vinegar to use is apple cider vinegar. Essential oils work very well with apple cider vinegar to tone the skin, cleanse the hair, and alkalinize the body.

aromatherapy for sensual living *steamy, dreamy, creamy: enthralling essential oil practices*

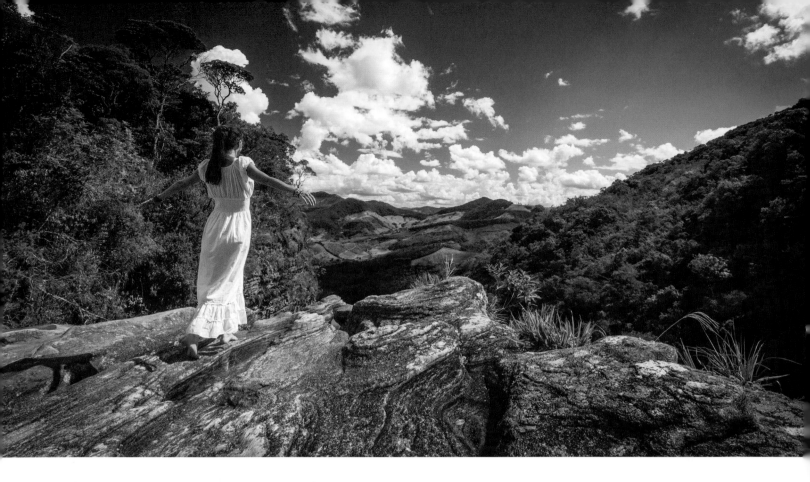

Aromatic Affirmations

As we claim and celebrate our innate sexy power, we empower ourselves in a deep, healthy, and loving way. That is the core of sensual living.

Your authentic sensual power (and the treasures that come with it) comes by digging in and committing to healing lifelong diminishing patterns. Luckily, you have essential oils on your side and they're brilliant activators, mood boosters, and sexy makers. There's genuine magic in those little bottles to help and heal.

To let my own sensuality bubble up to the surface, I practice a system called "aromatic affirmations" where I combine mantras and gentle self-massage and energy techniques along with essential oils. It's a powerful way to support the body, move through emotional sludge, and transcend. It's radiating beauty bliss available for you to practice anytime, anywhere.

When we combine our senses of sound, touch, and smell simultaneously, we amplify the speed of the healing process.

As you go through these affirmations, stay present to engage your senses while maintaining an even and steady breath. Sometimes, it only takes one session to change to a frequency that's more in line with your sensual mystique. More often, I recommend that my clients choose a maximum of three mantras and commit to doing them 108 times for 40 days.

Why affirmations?

Words have powerful vibrations. In Dr. Emoto's experiments, he showed that water molecules change their shape depending on what's written on a jar of water. Words like "love," "gratitude," and "peace" form beautiful crystalline formations, whereas words like "hate," "war," and "destruction" form irregular and disfigured shapes. Since we're made from mostly water, we can encode our bodies with messages that are dynamic, empowering, and love-filled.

In dark moments, we tend to forget that we have the ability to shape our daily experience. We can choose love or fear in every situation. Choose love.

Repeat your chosen affirmation slowly and with intention. Allow the potency of the oils to penetrate deeply inside of you. Track them. Ask for messages, clarity, and clearing on specific matters that are affecting your life. Keep a journal to record any memories, ideas, thoughts, or insights that come from this meditation. Perfumes have tremendous wisdom and healing ability. The more you welcome them in, the more they're able to work their magic.

Mind *Affirmation*

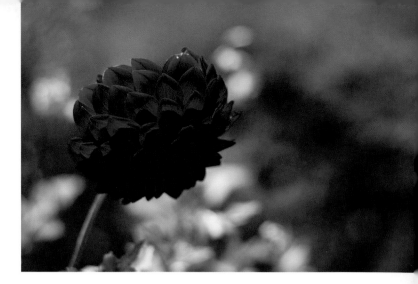

Non-beneficial thoughts can prevent us from moving forward into authentic action in our lives. Rise above them. Don't give those dark thoughts your vital energy; it will only drag you down and you have too much vibrant living to do.

This mantra clears the mental cobwebs to create quantifiable momentum into the life that you've always dreamed.

Add one drop of rosemary, black spruce, basil, or lemongrass to your fingertips. Place them on top of your head, your third eye, and at the base of your skull. Apply firm but gentle pressure to the head and state one of these affirmations:

"My thoughts are clear, focused, and supporting me to achieve my most intimate aspirations."

"I'm in full alignment with my higher and lower selves to create union, momentum, and perfect unfoldment."

"I trust my inner wisdom and use it to guide me in all aspects of life."

"I am present in this moment."

Throat *Chakra*

This affirmation can be done in two ways. You can pour one or two drops of oil over both hands and place them over your throat or eat one teaspoon of honey with one drop of oil. Take small servings of the honey/oil combination in your mouth and let it slowly melt. Sweet oil dripping over your vocal cords and throat is a seriously erotic experience. The essential oils that I like to use to tone and open the throat chakra are cape chamomile, steam-distilled benzoin, frankincense, and cypress.

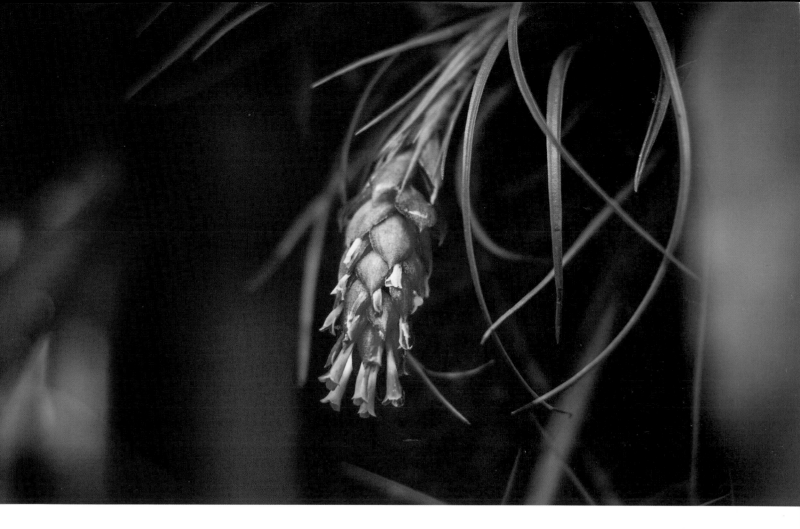

State these affirmations:

"My voice speaks the truth of love. Only love comes from my lips."

"I'm clear. I'm understood. I'm heard. I'm valued for what I have to say."

"I'm able to communicate my emotions effectively. I'm confident in my vulnerability."

Heart *Affirmation*

Love can be complicated for many women. Slowly but surely, we're learning to nurture our worth and voice our needs. Go, lady, go! You create the love you want in your life by nourishing the love you have in yourself. Be firm in love.

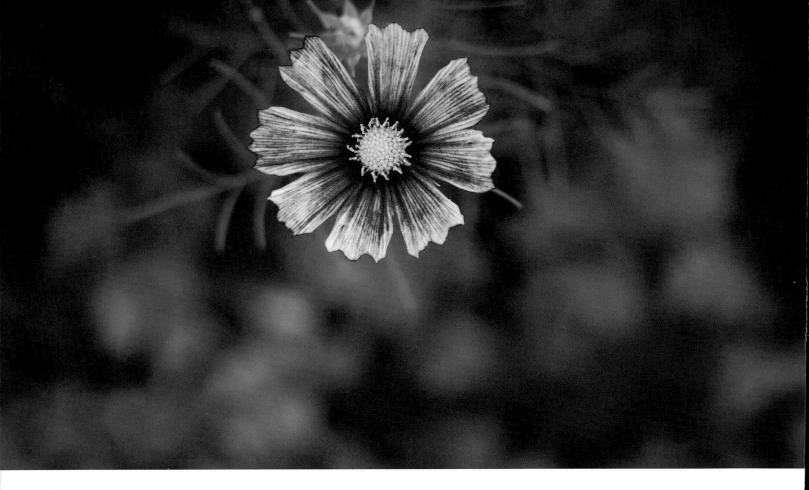

Add one drop of geranium, marjoram, or rose otto to the palm of your left hand and fingertips of your right hand. Place your left hand over your heart and your right hand over your sacral plexus (located two to three inches below your belly button) and state:

"My heart is a resilient, powerful organ whose purpose is to love and open fully. Only that which serves love is welcome in this space."

"I'm open to give and receive love."

"I completely love and accept myself and take regular action to support that love."

"I say yes and I am here."

Solar *Plexus Affirmation*

We store a lot of our emotional slop in our stomach area (the solar plexus). It's the bundle of nerves on the mid-line of the body that sits three inches below the sternum. The solar plexus controls the flight or fight response. It gives us momentum to move our lives forward and thrive in the place of self-respect and authentic confidence. Essential oils work beautifully to tone the solar plexus and are excellent confidence enhancers.

Anoint the palms of both hands with lemon, lemongrass, cypress, juniper berry, ginger, and/or fennel. With your left hand on your heart and your right hand on your solar plexus, state with conviction:

"I have the power within myself to create a meaningful, beautiful, rich life. I believe in myself."

"I'm at peace with myself and with the entire universe. Everything is flowing perfectly and in divine flow. I trust myself and my unfolding."

"I stand up for myself and believe in my personal power and worth."

Yoni *Affirmation*

Add one drop of rose otto, ylang ylang, geranium, sandalwood, cape chamomile, or C02 jasmine

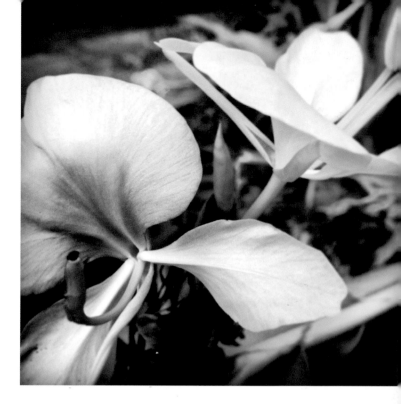

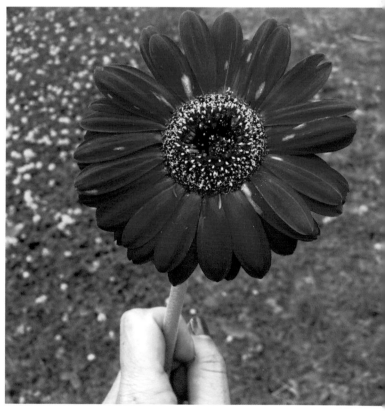

137

aromatherapy for sensual living *aromatic affirmations*

essential oil to the fingertips of both hands. With the gentlest touch, place both hands on your yoni petals to cover them entirely and state: "My body is a temple. I allow only love into this holy space."

This mantra helps those who suffered sexual abuse or aren't honoring themselves in their sexual relationships. Essential oils can remind you of your worth and beauty, if perhaps you've lost them on your way.

Other mantras or affirmations that are very effective for enlivening the yonis are:

- "My body opens to sacred, connected touch and is ready to receive it."

- "I'm grounded and feel safe in my world."

- "All of my needs are taken care of. I can rest and watch the unfolding of all my manifestations."

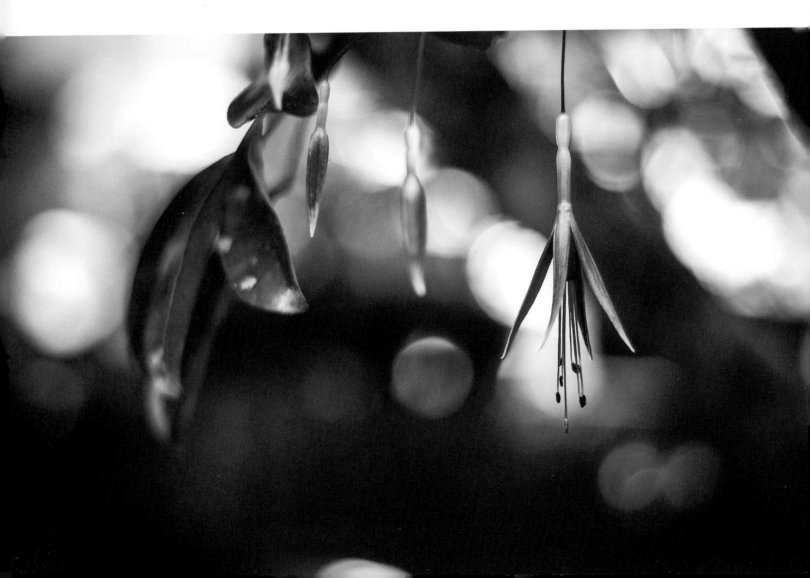

- "I'm worthy of respect, commitment, and consistent love, and I watch how it regularly shows up in my life."

"Go within yourself and out of your own self, fetch knowledge. You are the greatest book that ever was and ever will be, the infinite custodian of everything that is. All external teaching is vain so long as the inner teacher does not awake. It must cause the book of the heart to be open if it is to be of value."

– Swami Vivikanada

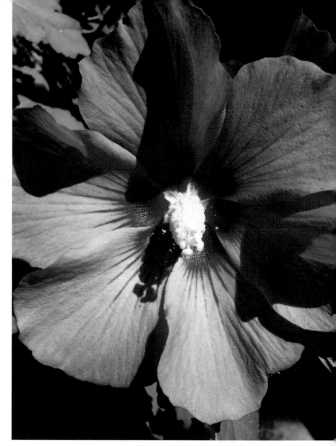

The *Sensual Force in Nature*

The sensual force is a pulsating currency that exists in nature and only increases its vibrancy as we open to the interconnectedness of life. It's by being present to all of our senses that we become awake, aware, and alive for the here and now of living. It's our juju juice in action. We just have to tune in.

Let your body ripple and succumb to its force. There are endless ways to fall into the rapture of nature and let it leave you breathless. Let it in. Its warm summer wind is blowing sweet nothings

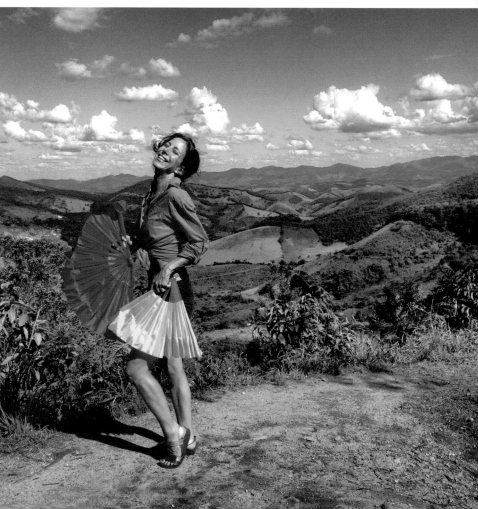

all over your skin, the knee-buckling beauty of cherry blossoms in full bloom or the rich smells of fallen autumn leaves. Nature is sexy everywhere. You just have to open your eyes and inhale. It's a beauty blessing.

Essential oils serve as a beautiful opener to awaken to the sensual force. They bring in the here and now.

Edible, Delectable, Downright Erotic: Essential Oils in the Kitchen

Food and sex are virtually inseparable. Have you ever purred audibly from eating a deep and delicious chocolate mousse? Have you ever ached for a flaky French croissant so deeply that you interrupted all your other plans in hot pursuit of your edible lover? I confess I have and I'm sure I will again. Food tempts our palates and satisfies us in a way that can be downright erotic.

We need food for survival as much as we need delicious bedroom romps. Food is utterly sensual as it engages all of our senses. How we nourish our bodies directly relates to how we honor our body temple and our connection to the divine. It's pretty exciting to feel sexy inspiration and holy communion from a bowl of sprouts with pumpkin seeds or a decadent red velvet cupcake.

In traditional Chinese medicine, the heart and the stomach are paired organs, meaning they work together to create harmony in the body. The way to a man's heart is through his stomach is undeniably true. I would add that the way to a man's passion is through his nose. If you smell good, he'll want you. A pleasing aroma leaves a lasting impression that tickles the sensual centers in the brain. That's potent flower power.

People are often surprised that most essential oils are edible and delicious. Many essential oil books chide the use of essential oils internally. I wholeheartedly encourage you to savor essential oils in moderation, with a maximum of 10 drops over a 24-hour period. They're an indispensable part of my daily sensual and health-care practice — with great results. Because essential oils are antibacterial, antifungal, and antimicrobial, they're also my health-boosting tool of choice.

If you use essential oils in food, make sure they are from a reputable company, steam-distilled or CO_2-extracted. Most culinary oils are steam-distilled, so if you have the raw herb, flower, or bark in your kitchen, chances are you can use the essential oils for culinary purposes as well. Most tree oils are steam-distilled and make a welcome addition to any spirited drink or salad dressing. Please don't consume bay laurel, nutmeg, wintergreen, or clary sage, as they have unwanted narcotic effects.

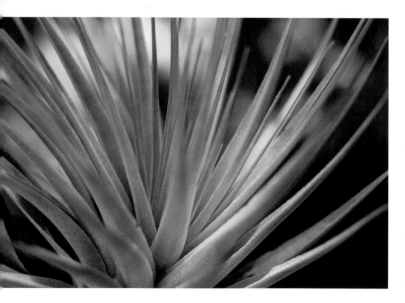

Essential oils can easily take over any dish. Please refer to the section on pouring principles. A steady and patient hand is what you need to ensure that you don't mistakenly drop more than you intend. Keep the bottle at eye level. The secret is in the pour.

Aromatherapy and food make for a playground of creativity and ingenuity. I have often used a drop of rosemary or thyme linalool if I'm out of the raw herb and want to intensify the flavor of a dish. There are endless flavor combinations to use, and all of them are exciting. Let your creativity come to life.

aromatherapy for sensual living *edible, delectable, downright erotic: essential oils in the kitchen*

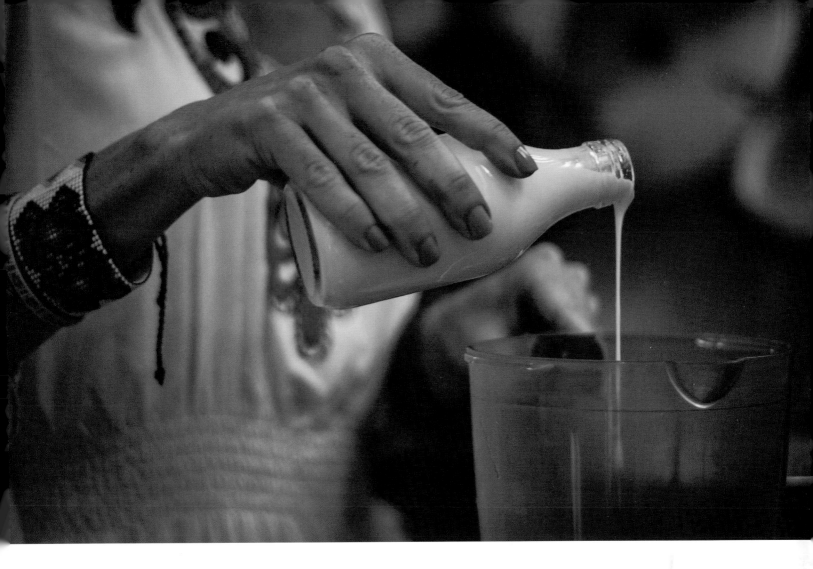

Essential oils gravitate toward sweet foods like fruits, honey, maple syrup, stevia, agave, or any kind of fat like olive oil, coconut oil, ghee, hemp seeds, avocado, or pumpkin seed oil. If your recipe calls for one of these ingredients, feel confident knowing that essential oils will combine easily and be utterly delightful.

Essential oils break down with light, heat, and air. If you're adding essential oils to hot food, please do so at the very end or once the food has cooled slightly to maximize the flavor and strength of the oils. For all of their potency, they're surprisingly delicate. Don't let that stop you from experimenting. The more you use essential oils, the more places you will find to incorporate them into your life and lifestyle. The result will be a stronger and more vital immune system, beauty from the inside out, and unforgettable meals and treats.

Juices

Juicing is a fantastic way to amp your health and vitality. I tend to enjoy vegetable juices over fruit juices because of the high sugar content in fruit juice, though there's a time and place for everything. Here are some of my favorite aromatic juices.

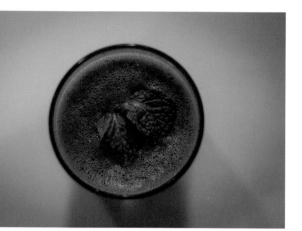

Watermelon *Thirst Quencher*

Watermelon is a marvelous summer treat. I love to dilute it with coconut water in order to reduce the sugar content and deepen the nutritional content. Watermelon is an excellent way to detox the kidneys and adrenals. Avoid food two hours before or after eating watermelon.

Use:

- 3 cups of watermelon, including seeds

- 1 cup of raw, unpasteurized coconut water

- 1 drop of immortelle

Combine all of the ingredients in a high-speed blender. Garnish with a small mint leaf. Serve immediately. With this drink, it's best to avoid other foods for three hours to ensure easy digestion.

Serves 4

Papaya *Juice with Coconut and Vanilla (With Seeds)*

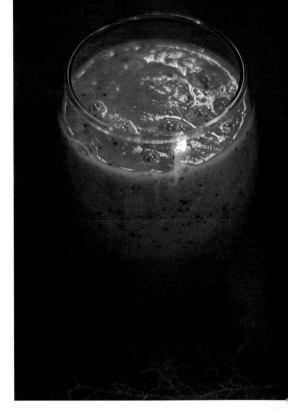

Papaya is an outstanding fruit. It contains enzymes called papain that effectively aid digestion. The seeds are also an effective anti-parasitic cleanse. I use half the seeds in my shake. They impart a sharp peppery taste that can be unusual for some, but I find it delicious.

Use:

- ½ large papaya or 2 or 3 small ones

- ¾ cup organic coconut milk

- ½ cup of spring water

- 1 drop of vanilla essential oil

Blend all of the ingredients together in a high-speed blender. Garnish with a sprinkle of vanilla powder and serve. This dreamy drink will cause you to float away on a coconut cloud of bliss. Bring your lover, too.

Serves 2–3

Cucumber *Cooling Cocktail*

Cucumbers internally cool the body in intense summer heat. Adding the smallest pinch of sea salt will open up the cell wall to further hydrate the cell. Combined with peppermint, this is a sparkling summer hydrating treat that will soon be your favorite.

Use:

- 1 organic English cucumber

- 2 cups of raw organic coconut water

- 1 small handful of flat-leaf parsley

- 1 drop of peppermint essential oil

- 1 pinch of Himalayan sea salt

Blend all of the ingredients together in a high-speed blender. Serve immediately with a sprig of parsley. It's guaranteed to freshen the breath, too.

Serves 4

Love *Me Tender Pink Rose Petal Lemonade*

Lemons simply squeal for the sweet petaled treasure of rose. It's a harmonic combination that's both delicious and beautiful. Lemons are wonderful astringents for the kidneys, support detoxification pathways, and help to alkalize the body. Roses are a pure and loving salve for the heart and loins.

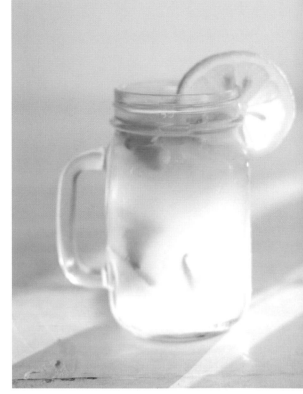

Use:

- 4–6 squeezed lemons, making one cup of lemon juice

- 4–6 tablespoons of raw organic honey (to taste)

- 1 small organic, de-petaled pink rose head

- 4 cups of spring water

- 1–3 drops of rose otto

- 1 handful of ice

- Optional: a splash of rose syrup

Combine the honey with one cup of water in a saucepan and cook on low heat to make simple syrup. Stir until combined. Add all the ingredients except the rose petals and ice to a high-speed blender. Blend. Strain if necessary. Add the rose petals and ice and stir well. Serve immediately. Adorn with a sprig of mint.

Serves 4

aromatherapy for sensual living *edible, delectable, downright erotic: essential oils in the kitchen*

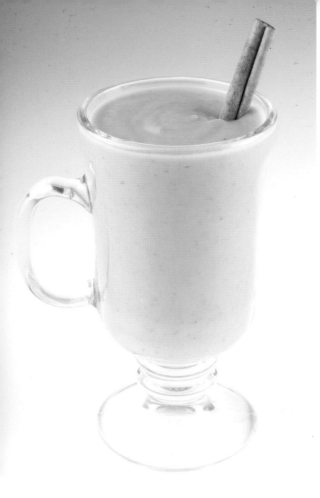

Hot *Sweet Potato Shake*

This shake is unbelievably delicious and perfect for a cold winter day. It's warm and nourishing with just the right amount of sweetness. It makes a wonderful breakfast or a deeply satisfying midday snack. Cinnamon is an all-over body warmer. This shake is sensual delight that tingles from your toes to the top of your head.

Use:

- 2 medium-sized sweet potatoes

- ½ cup of organic coconut milk

- 1–2 cups of water to reach desired thickness

- 1 drop of cinnamon essential oil

Boil the sweet potatoes covered in shallow water for 15 minutes or steam them for 30 minutes in a bamboo steamer. Check the water often to make sure that there's enough in the pot. Once cooked, discard the peel. Add a half cup of coconut milk along with two cups of hot water to a high-speed blender. Add one drop of cinnamon.

Serves 2

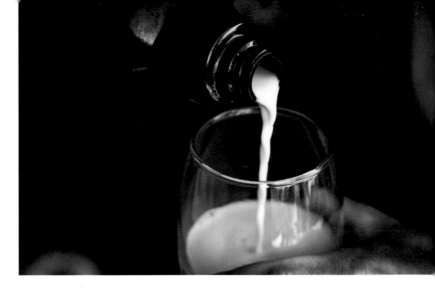

Almond *Milk*

Almond milk is a creamy and delicious delight. Once you try homemade almond milk, you might never go back to the chemical-laden, pasteurized, store-bought variety. Almond milk is rich in protein and can be used in place of other milks in cooking or enjoyed on its own. The addition of cardamom makes this milk supremely sensual and warming in all the right places.

Use:

- 1 cup of organic, unpasteurized almonds

- 2 medjool dates

- 3 cups of spring water and soaking water

- 1 drop of cardamom or vanilla essential oil

Cover and soak almonds in spring water for 6–12 hours. Discard the soaking water. Add fresh water, almonds, dates, and cardamom or vanilla essential oil to a high-speed blender for one to two minutes. Pour the mixture through a cheesecloth or preferably a nut milk bag with a large bowl underneath. Squeeze the nut milk through the bag until no liquid remains and the almond mixture is dry to the touch. Enjoy your milk for up to three days.

Save the pulverized nuts for a side recipe. You can use them as alternative baking flour, a high-protein addition to your breakfast porridge, garnish for soups and more.

Serves 3

Breakfast

Sweet Relief Breakfast Porridge

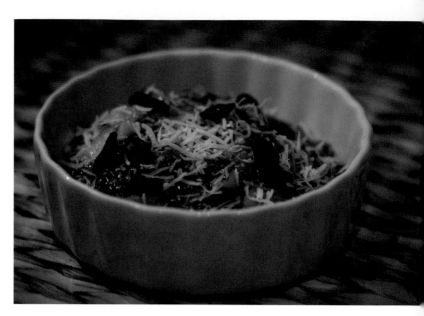

There's something deeply satisfying about stewed fruit on a cold winter morning. The combination of chia and fruit helps for easy digestion and morning yumminess that's totally addictive. In my clinic, I say: "Better out than in." This recipe ensures easy bowel motility and the added benefit of a clear mind, steady emotions, radiant skin, a flatter tummy, and a stronger immune system.

Use:

- 1 tablespoon of whole chia soaked at a ten-to-one ratio in water

- 1 cup of organic granola

- 1 cup of organic milk or almond milk

- ½ cup of stewed apples

- 1 tablespoon of coconut flakes

- 1 drop of fenugreek essential oil

- pomegranates and berries are optional

Stewed Apples

- 2 chopped apples

- 1 tablespoon of coconut oil

aromatherapy for sensual living *edible, delectable, downright erotic: essential oils in the kitchen*

- 1 zested orange

- ½ teaspoon each of cinnamon, cardamom, and vanilla powder (essential oils also work well)

- 4 tablespoons of water

- pinch of salt

- 1 teaspoon of maple syrup or honey is optional

Chop two apples into bite-sized pieces. Put them in a frying pan on medium heat with coconut oil or ghee, water, cinnamon, vanilla, cardamom, and orange zest. Allow the apples to cook down for a minimum of twenty minutes and up to forty minutes. Stir often.

Combine the granola, stewed apples, coconut shavings, chia, and additional fruit in a separate bowl. Serve immediately.

Serves 2

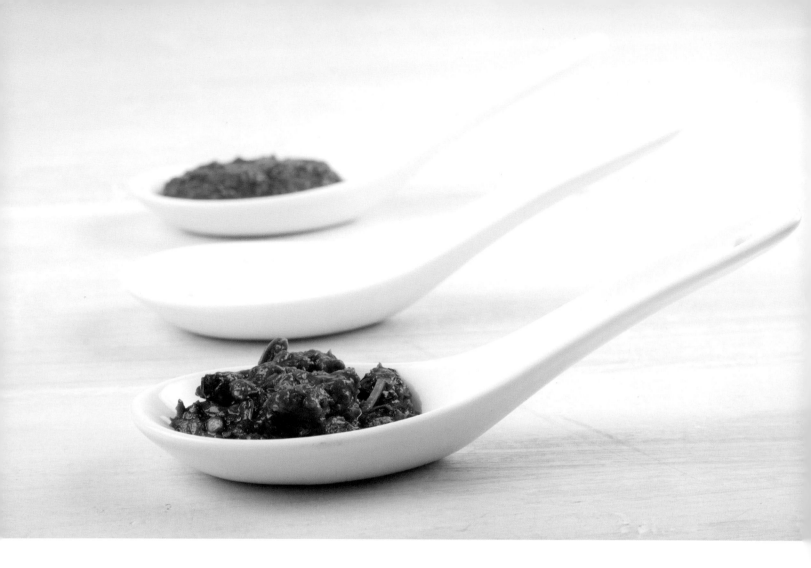

Sauces *and Spreads*

Bright Sauce

Use:

- 1 cup of soaked, raw and peeled cashews or almonds

- ½ cup of homemade, unsweetened almond milk

- ½ cup of olive oil

- 1 clove of garlic

- 1 tablespoon of grainy Dijon mustard

- ½ lemon, juiced and zested

- 1 tablespoon of apple cider vinegar

- 1 teaspoon of turmeric powder or essential oil

- salt to taste

- 1 drop each of thyme linalool, tarragon, rosemary and sage oil

Add everything except olive oil to a high-speed blender. Blend until unified. Slowly drip olive oil into the blender at a medium high speed to emulsify the sauce. Add additional almond milk or olive oil to reach the desired creaminess. It's called bright sauce because it makes everything come alive with a blast of turmeric-infused color.

Serve with crunchy bread, avocados, thinly sliced shallots, tomatoes, arugula, radishes, and boiled quail eggs.

Punched-up *Pesto*

Green vegetables are nutritional powerhouses that make my insides sing. The benefits of green leafy vegetables include increased immunity; antioxidant properties; easing bowel motility; better brain function; and speeding recovery from an illness. I aim to eat at least one solid serving of green vegetables every day. Pesto is an easy way to get your greens. Just make sure you have a toothbrush handy. Those little suckers can hide in the corners of your teeth. The addition of rosemary oil lifts the greens and gives the pesto depth and an immune-boosting kick.

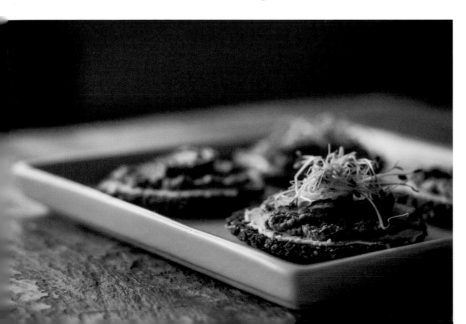

Use:

- 1 full head of washed and dried arugula

- 1 cup of walnuts, cashews or pine nuts that have soaked for 6 to 18 hours

- 1 clove of garlic

- ½ cup of olive oil

- pinch of salt

- 1–2 drops of rosemary oil

- sun dried tomatoes, hemp seeds, olives, and seaweed are options

Trim the arugula and wash off soiled spots. Chop the garlic and place it in a food processor, followed by the remainder of the ingredients except the olive oil. Blend until unified. Slowly add olive oil to the blender to emulsify the sauce, and continue to add oil to reach your desired creaminess.

Serve on whole-grain crackers topped with avocado, sundried tomatoes, goat cheese, and a crack of pepper. It can also be served on brown rice pasta, on top of roasted chicken, or on hot and crunchy bread. My personal favorite is a rice bowl with sprouts, avocado, dulse seaweed, sweet potatoes, and green onions.

Tapenade

If I had to choose between sweet and savory, I'd choose savory any day. Olives are perfect for satisfying that salty temptation. I like to keep a jar of them kicking around to spice up any meal or casual gathering. Black foods such as olives, according to traditional Chinese medicine, have the ability to super-charge your kidneys — the back-up batteries in the body. If you're feeling sluggish, slow, or sour, try to eat some salty food in moderation.

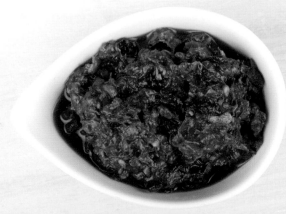

Use:

- 1 cup of pitted, organic black olives

- 2 tablespoons of drained capers

- 1 solid handful of fresh, lightly chopped parsley

- 8–10 cherry tomatoes or 1 large Roma tomato

- 1 teaspoon of fresh thyme or 1 tablespoon of dried thyme

- 2 tablespoons of olive oil

- 1 tablespoon of red wine vinegar

- ½ squeezed lemon

- 1–2 drops of thyme linalool oil

- 1 drop of sage oil

- solid pinch of Maldon salt

Add all of the ingredients to a food processor. Slowly add additional olive oil to achieve desired consistency. It will stay fresh for five days.

This recipe is just about perfect on whitefish, brown rice, crackers, or mixed into lentils.

Raw *Ketchup*

Once you've made your own ketchup, you'll never buy that sugary, synthetic, lasts-for-eternity-on-the-shelf variety again. This is the one your taste buds long for. It's fresh, deep, flavorful, delicious, and easy to make.

Use:

- 1 ½ cups of diced organic tomatoes

- 3 tablespoons of chopped dates

- ¼ cup of olive oil

- 1 teaspoon of sea salt

- 1 tablespoon of apple cider vinegar

- ½ cup of dry sun dried tomatoes

- 1 drop each of thyme linalool, rosemary, and tarragon oils

Blend everything except the sundried tomatoes in a high-speed blender. Add the sundried tomatoes last and blend until you get a ketchup consistency. Feel free to add olives to deepen the flavor profile.

Herbed *butters*

I positively love my fats. They provide long-lasting energy and satiety. Sadly, butter has been vilified as an artery-clogging, health-harming culprit for decades. But in truth, authentic natural fats are one of the best things you can put in your body. Moderation is the key. Butter is a natural source of vitamin K and long-chain saturated fats. Butter makes everything better.

Use:

- ½ pound of organic butter (salted or unsalted)

- 1 teaspoon of fresh flowers, such as calendula, violets, nasturtiums, sage flowers, rosemary flowers, or thyme flowers

- 1 drop of rosemary and sage oils

Allow butter to come to room temperature. Slowly add the flowers and essential oils. Store in an airtight container. Serve on potatoes, meat, rice, or anywhere where butter would do it better.

Soup *and Salad*

Gazpacho

Gazpacho is a fabulous and cooling summer soup. Essential oils will lend themselves easily to the flavor and body of the soup.

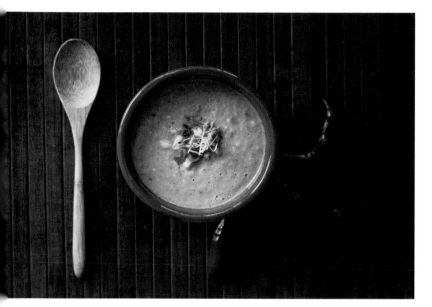

Use:

- 4 ripe tomatoes
- 1 finely chopped cucumber
- 1 finely chopped red onion or shallot
- 1 seeded and chopped sweet bell pepper
- 2 stalks of halved and chopped celery
- 2 tablespoons of chopped parsley
- 2 tablespoons of chopped cilantro
- 1 tablespoon of spring chives
- 1 clove of minced garlic
- ¼ cup of red wine or apple cider vinegar
- ¼ cup of olive oil
- juice from half a lemon
- 1 teaspoon of honey
- salt and pepper to taste
- 1 seeded and chopped serrano or jalapeno pepper
- 1 teaspoon of shoyu, tamari, or high quality soy sauce
- 1 drop each of black pepper, lemon, basil, and thyme linalool oils

Blend all of the ingredients in a high-speed blender to reach desired consistency. Reserve one table-spoon each of red onion, cucumber, and celery, as well as a pinch of parsley for a garnish. Store in a mason jar overnight to allow the flavors to meld and mingle. It's a delicious and aromatic summertime treat that's perfect with crusty bread drenched in an aromatic olive oil.

Vichyssoise

Sometimes the greatest thing in the world is a cold potato soup. While not glamorous, vichyssoise is utterly delicious and so satis-fying. The soup is made considerably more compelling with a single drop of tarragon essential oil.

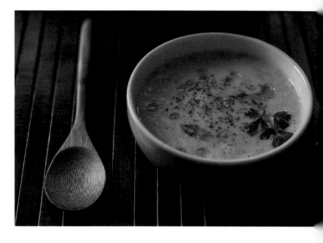

Use:

- 2 leeks chopped up to pale green section

- 1 large chopped shallot

- 2 tablespoons of unsalted butter or ghee

- ¾ cup of thinly sliced organic red potatoes

- 2 ⅓ cups of vegetarian or chicken stock

- 1 cup of heavy cream or unsweetened almond milk

- salt and pepper to taste

- 1 drop of tarragon essential oil

- 2 tablespoons of finely chopped parsley

- a shaving of nutmeg

Melt the butter or ghee in a large pot on medium low heat. Add onions and leeks and allow them to sweat slightly without allowing them to brown. Stir often for approximately 8 minutes. Add potatoes, stock, salt, and pepper to the saucepan. Bring to a gentle boil and simmer for 30 minutes. Puree soup in a high-speed blender until smooth. Allow it to cool. Add one drop of tarragon along with almond milk or heavy cream. Garnish with parsley. Enjoy.

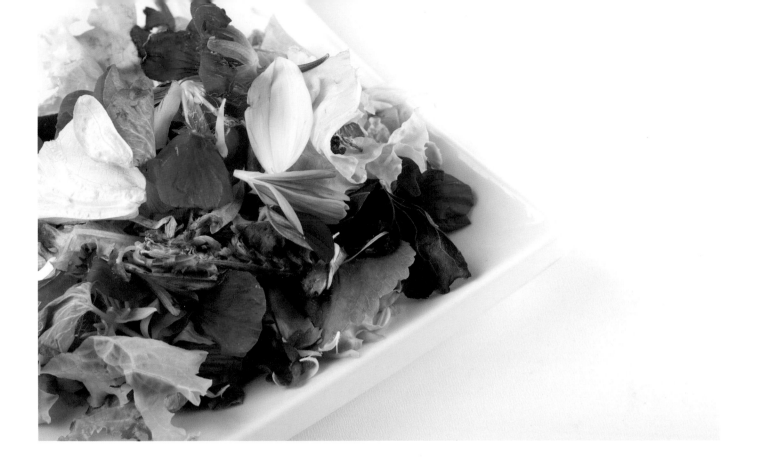

Wild Salad

Foraging for wild food is an awesome way to reconnect to nature and celebrate your untamed desire. I take giddy delight from being able to source food that's natural, nutritionally dense, and utterly potent in its flavor. Eating flowers is delightful. These are all great options for a wild salad:

- Purple chive heads

- Yellow dandelion heads

- Green-grey spruce tips

- Multi-color violets

- Chopped mint leaves

- Wild leeks

aromatherapy for sensual living   *edible, delectable, downright erotic: essential oils in the kitchen*

- Arugula

- Lamb's quarters

- Nasturtiums

- Calendula

- Rose petals

- Sage flowers

- Rosemary flowers

- Thyme flowers

Many of these might already be growing in your back yard and if not, grow them in your garden or in pots on your balcony. You can experiment with other wild food like wild mushrooms too.

Mix together a wild salad. For a salad dressing, add a drop of Mediterranean salad oil along with olive oil, apple cider vinegar, one teaspoon of honey, and a pinch of salt. Blend well and serve.

Essential Herb Oils

I keep a bottle of this oil blend in my kitchen to amp up the flavor quotient at the end of cooking. One drop is perfect to enhance the flavor of any meal. It can be used in hummus, meats, salad dressings, and omelets. It's delicious and utterly easy to use.

Add 10 to 20 drops of each oil in a 50-milliliter bottle. Add organic olive oil to the top. Store in a cool and dark place. Conversely, you can make a blend from the essential oils listed below and add drops to an existing bottle of olive oil until you reach your desired potency.

- Mediterranean: thyme linalool, rosemary, basil, oregano, tarragon, mastic

- Indian: cinnamon, cardamom, ginger, cumin, coriander, black pepper, fenugreek

- Thai: lemongrass, lime, tarragon

Dessert

Tropical Mango Sorbet

Mango is one of the most sensual, dripping, and delicious fruits. They're also a great source of vitamin A and are alkalizing to the body. Though this recipe is slightly labor-intensive, it's totally worth it. A lot of the work can be alleviated by using an ice cream maker.

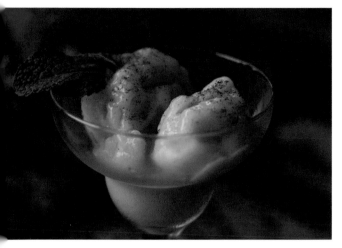

Use:

- 4 large and ripe mangos
- 1 cup of simple syrup made with half a cup of honey and half a cup of water
- juice from 1 lime plus zest
- 1 drop of vanilla or cardamom essential oil
- ½ cup of full fat coconut milk is optional

Stand the mangoes upright and cut them on either side of the seed to slice them in two. Score the mangoes in a checkerboard pattern. Fold them inside out and use a soup spoon to scoop out the flesh.

Add the mangoes, simple syrup, lime, vanilla, and coconut milk to a high-speed blender for a few minutes.

Transfer to a freezer-proof dish (metal is preferred). Fold the mango puree every 45 minutes for 4 hours to keep it from freezing into a large mango ice cube. After 4 hours, allow the sorbet to sit in the freezer for 8 hours. Eat and enjoy.

Serves 4

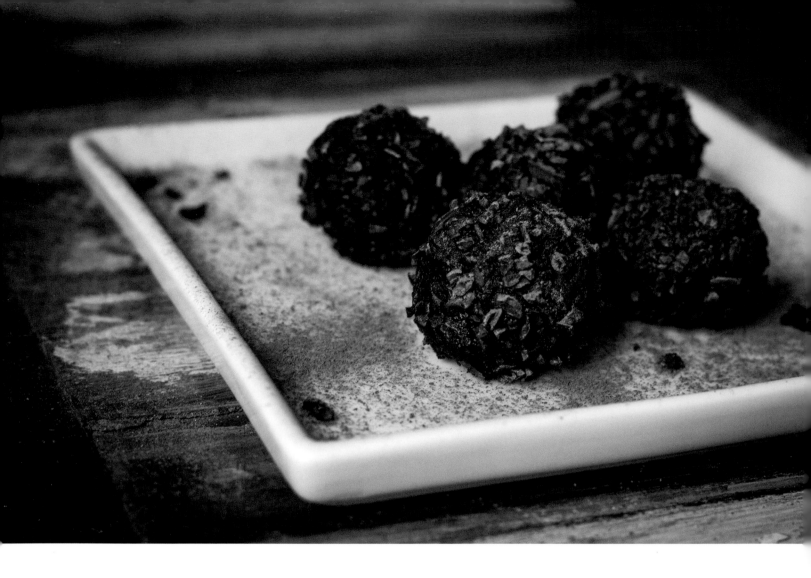

Salty Chocolate Balls

I make these energy bombs for exercise marathons or long walks in the woods. You never know when you're going to need a little energy pick-me-up on your path. Chocolate is known to induce dopamine (the pleasure molecule) in the brain. With a rush of dopamine, our bodies feel like we're falling in love. Raw cacao also has the highest level of magnesium of any food. Magnesium is the molecule responsible for relaxation in the body, and most people are magnesium deficient. Raw cacao helps everything feel good, right, and downright dreamy. Combined with essential oils, it's a guaranteed bliss trip to ecstasy.

aromatherapy for sensual living   *edible, delectable, downright erotic: essential oils in the kitchen*

Combine these ingredients in a food processor in order, pulsing in between:

- 1 cup of raw pumpkin seeds

- ¾ cup of organic goji berries

- 8–12 pitted organic dates (more to taste)

- 1 ¼ cups of raw cacao powder

- 1 tablespoon of vanilla powder

- ½ cup of raw, organic coconut oil

- ½ cup of rice bran powder

- ½ tablespoon of Maldon sea salt flakes

- 1 drop of cardamom, cinnamon, clove, tarragon, fenugreek, ginger, or thyme essential oil, or orange rind or organic rose petals. Use your imagination. Chocolate tastes good with so many things.

Roll the mixture into one-inch balls. If the coconut oil is liquid (due to summer heat or a hot kitchen), place it in the fridge for 15 minutes to firm up. Feel free to play with the amounts to personalize your salty chocolate balls to taste. Store in a sealed container lined with wax paper. They'll keep for five days on the counter or two weeks in the fridge.

Makes approximately 24 balls.

Essential oils in food impart a potent flavor quotient to any edible treat. They also transfer medicinal, immune-boosting, antibacterial, and anti-parasitic properties right into your stomach and all other organs. It's a disco dance party for your taste buds and lymphatic immune system. I've been using essential oils as flavor enhancers and immune stimulants for twenty years and haven't had to use western suppressive medicine.

Make Your Own Incense

Most incense is a toxic pool of allergy-inducing garbage. It makes me cough, sneeze, and want to leave the room immediately. Sensual lovers — in an effort to imbibe what's authentic, euphoric, and ecstatic — I invite you to make your own. It's not difficult, and there's something ancient and even magical about making incense. I make a lot at once as it's rather time-intensive. Use a powerful high-speed blender or sturdy pestle and mortar to finely chop the herbs and resins.

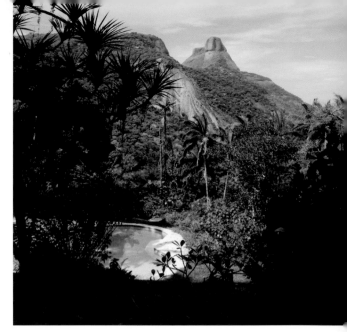

Use:

- A variety of fragrant herbs such as resins: frankincense, myrrh, copal, copaiba, dragon's blood, mastic, galbanum, agar wood, aloeswood

- Spices: vanilla, star anise, cinnamon, vanilla, cardamom

- Herbs: patchouli, roses, sweetgrass, deer's tongue, melilot, tonka, jasmine, lavender, yellow sandalwood

- A mortar and pestle

- Arabic gum

- Charcoal tablets

- A small amount of water

- Creative flair

Place arabic gum in a small bowl. Slowly add water drop by drop until the mixture has a gummy-like quality. If you add too much water, your incense won't hold together. If you don't add enough, it will crumble and fall apart. It should have the consistency of molasses. Let it sit for three hours while you pulverize the herbs. I tend to use no more than five kinds of herbs in the mix and generally stick to two or three.

Slowly add your herb combination to the solidified arabic gum. Form the incense into a variety of shapes. Try shaping your incense with a definable tip like a cone or pyramid so the heat can burn the incense down evenly. You can also try rolling your incense into thin tubes and inserting a thin, pliable stick of wood. You can often find appropriate sticks in Chinese stores.

Allow your formed incense to dry for 24 hours before burning. The simplest way to burn incense is to get an empty jar, cover the lid with aluminum foil, and carefully poke holes into the aluminum foil with a tip of a fork. Light the charcoal tablet. Once it has caught, place the incense on top of the charcoal tablet on the aluminum foil. The air underneath the foil will help the incense to burn entirely without having to relight it. Another option is to place it on an electric stove top, burn the tip of the incense, and place it on a fire-proof plate. With this method, however, you'll have to continually relight.

Incense is amazing for many reasons. Of course it makes your home smell naturally divine but, more than that, incense has been used for centuries to fumigate stagnant places, remove unwanted energies, or energetically clean a space. It's powerful what a little smoke can do for a room.

If you're feeling stuck, anxious, depressed, or angry, try fumigating your home. Make sure you leave a window open so all that negative energy has a place to go.

Keep your incense in a sealed container away from heat, light, and air. It can keep for years if stored properly, and it makes a fantastic and unique gift.

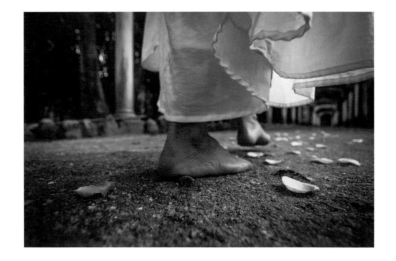

aromatherapy for sensual living   *edible, delectable, downright erotic: essential oils in the kitchen*

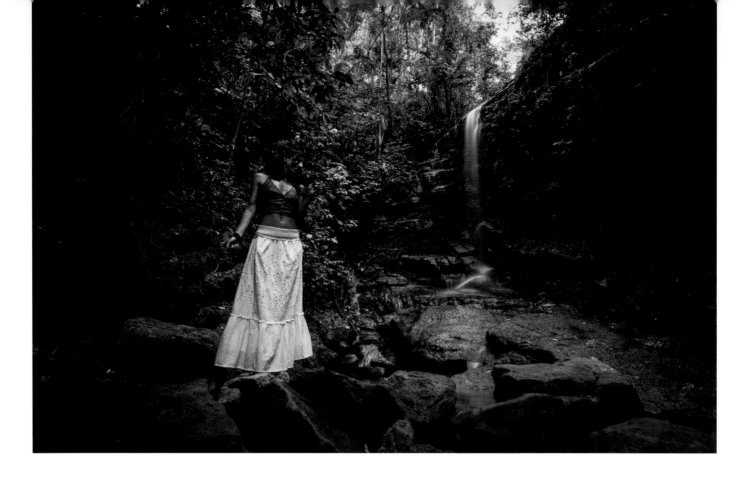

Deepening *Sensuality: Discover Your Aromatic Inspiration*

Through my lifelong aromatic affair, I've had many twists and turns as to what inspires me aromatically. It's good to deeply dive into one aroma for a period of time in order to learn its unique signature and capabilities. In my early twenties, I was positively charmed by ylang ylang. I used it every day for about a year and a half. I just couldn't get enough of that exotic, sensual, and intoxicating scent.

Part of my fascination was that I read (and confirmed) that ylang ylang is a powerful aphrodisiac. Ylang ylang is a vixen. It powerfully calms shock, eases menstrual cramps, and acts like a loving and supportive friend. Its power can be overwhelming to those who aren't accustomed to the aromatic dominance of certain flowers. I've since softened my desire to be so fragrantly forceful. Ah, the pleasures and foolishness of youth.

After ylang ylang, I started playing with circulatory oils like juniper berry, cypress, black pepper, and lemongrass. I was slightly rounder at that time and used these oils to help break down stubborn cellulite. One night I bathed in hot water, sea salt, and three potent circulation essential oils and then covered my body in a 30 percent circulatory oil blend with jojoba. The result was intense and palpable. My breath quickened, I was hyper-alert (it was close to midnight), and I could feel the oils pumping through my system to clear out unwanted stagnation. I had seen the light. I then focused my energy to make salt scrubs and cleaning products with these oils for my clients.

I later moved on to tree oils and found a grounding, ascension, and opening for the mind and lungs that I'd been aching for, without realizing it! Tree oils are purposeful and gentle in their way. Everyone feels good in the forest as we benefit from the negative ions released in verdant green spaces.

Tree oils are effective for city-dwellers who are unable to luxuriate in nature's playground. With one whiff, you can be instantly transported to a virgin British Columbia forest, rich with red cedars, or arrive in a somber Russian forest saturated with black spruce trees. Tree oils help me remember to stand tall, be firm, and remain beautiful despite life's winds of change. Most men seem to embrace to tree oils.

I'm now deeply into euphorics, which isn't surprising considering the theme of this book. Sandalwood, neroli, jasmine, vanilla, cape chamomile, ylang ylang, ginger, cinnamon, cacao, tarragon, and fenugreek make me melt, swoon, and soar. They're evocative and inspiring in countless ways. I recommend digging deep into euphorics for a lengthy period like I did with ylang ylang. However, it's not just for hot and steamy nights. It's a way to feel the flowers and allow them to lift you up out of whatever non-sparkly mood you're in. They make you high; not in a stoner hippie kind of way, but one that is elevated, enhanced, and more colorful. They're wonderful for connecting with a lover and making things all the more blushing.

Some people are attracted to deep and heavy base notes. Others like heady and dewy floral notes. There are those who prefer delightful and energetic citrus aromas. It's all good, healing, immune-supportive, and delicious. Trust that your scent preferences will vary through life experience and hormonal changes. There's so much abundance and variety that it's virtually impossible to get bored.

Your unique smell combination helps to shape and inform others of your personality, vitality, and sensuality. Sometimes you might be a scent siren with tuberose, jasmine, and vanilla. In a more buoyant moment, you might sport cypress, rosemary, and lemon. By deeply imbibing essential oils, you'll bathe your cells in the powerful, perfumed, and medicinal qualities of the plants and take them into your being and very soul. The question is: What colorful, delicious, and intoxicating aromatic message do you want to put out there?

Smell is tied to memory. When you use a particular scent, people will remember you and your unique essence. With essential oils, you can make your personal aroma natural, fantastic, exciting, alluring, and unforgettable. I am constantly being told, with a purr and sometimes a wink, that people often remember me years later because of the way I smell. I do love leaving that impression.

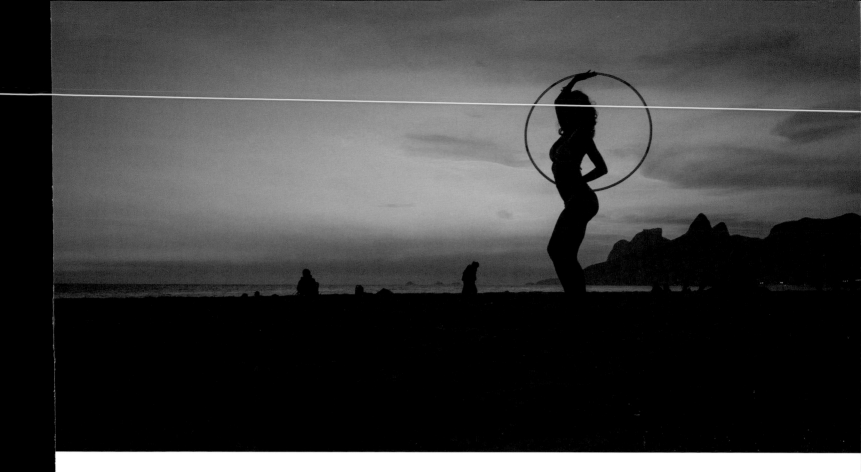

The Scented Diary

Dear aroma diary:

I'm meeting Captain Fantastic tonight and feeling all kinds of butterflies and sparkles. He is so dreamy with his piercing green eyes and strong, capable arms. I have a feeling it's going to be a very special night. My plan is to saturate myself in provocative erotic oils. I'm going to use a variety of essential oil combinations. Covering myself from head to toe in silky and sensual aromatherapy enriches my whole body with the potent power of plants and, tonight, I want to pulsate. Oh I blush.

I'm starting with a facial steam infused with neroli and rose hydrosol to open my pores and extract all the unnecessary grime that lies beneath the skin, followed by a mud mask enriched with skin-softening essential oils like sandalwood, rose otto, geranium, frankincense, and cape chamomile. I'll wash off the mask, spray my face with rose hydrosol, and allow it to dry. Finally, I'll anoint my face with rich and healing oils and massage them in deeply and lovingly.

I'm doing a deep conditioning treatment on my hair with warmed jojoba and coconut oil infused with rosemary. That will definitely help circulation and mental force. I'll let the hair treatment sit for twenty minutes and, in that time, I'll sugar scrub my hands and feet with ginger, grapefruit, and lemongrass. I want my feet to be oh-so-touchable, as I hope there's a foot massage in store for me later. Captain Fantastic is great with his hands.

Before I get in the shower, I'll dry brush my entire body slowly and deliberately, starting at the feet and moving up to the heart to circulate my lymph and remove dead and dry skin. I'll add drops of laurel, cypress, and lemon to the brush to boost circulation and help move stagnant lymph and have endlessly touchable skin. Dry brushing is an excellent way to make that happen.

I'll slowly, lovingly wash and condition my hair in the shower, being sure to pull the hair at the root. A well-timed, deliberate hair tug is magnetic and sends shivers all the way down my spine. I'll massage my head deeply, finding the little nooks and crannies where I'm holding tension. I'll spend extra time on these spots as an act of simple self-love. I'll shave because I love the feeling of soft skin touching my silk dress, not because society tells women that they need to be hairless. I'll use a natural soap blended with cape chamomile and sandalwood to soothe my sensitive skin.

I'll spend at least twenty minutes after my shower massaging and body-oiling every part of me with jojoba, coconut oil, cacao butter, jasmine, immortelle, grapefruit, and lavender. I'll send love and intention into every sweep and motion. Touching my body with the possibility of things to come is endlessly exciting.

I'll dab cape chamomile, tansy, rose otto, and lavender diluted in jojoba around my eyes. The azure tones of the oils help to calm inflammation, puffy eyes, and dark circles. I definitely want my blue eyes to sparkle.

My lady petals will be vibrant once they are anointed with jojoba and only the softest essential oils. That alone will plump me up and make me eager for his invited touch. I have to remember to pop some in my purse for later. It's good to have it around before and after the graceful union. And, oh my, it feels so good to be dappled down there.

I'll rub enticing and erotic essential oils like jasmine or tuberose through my hair. I have to be extra careful to only use one drop. Too much of a good thing can quickly turn into a bad thing. I want just enough so the fragrance blooms through our time together. Oils in the hair can last for two to three days.

Once completely oiled, I'll resist the temptation to put on clothes immediately. I'll stand naked to appreciate my body. It's vitally important and something that is usually rushed. I want to take my time today. I want to commune profoundly feeling its power, calming any pre-date nerves and infusing my body with deep and nutritive healing. In my naked time, I appreciate my unique beauty and body in a way that informs confidence and self-love.

I think I'll sneak out and lie in the sun since it's an incredible activator in so many ways. A boost of vitamin D is a guaranteed happy-maker.

Once out of the sun, I'll put on my dress. I'll anoint my armpits with sandalwood deodorant and spray delicious perfume on all my hot spots: the neck, wrists, inner elbows, upper inner thighs, behind the knees, and at the ankles. This man has no idea the treats that lie in store for him.

I want to make sure that he feels comfortable when he's here. I'm going to make a room spray of tangerine, hay, and magnolia blossom to lift his spirits and calm his soul. Fenugreek, lavender, vanilla, and sandalwood would also work well, but tangerine is always his favorite. I'm also going to put quite a few drops of vanilla and grapefruit in the front foyer so he knows he's being met by an ascended aromatic experience. It's simply irresistible.

Now to the kitchen . . .

Captain Fantastic deserves an aromatic feast. I'll start with spring water infused with vanilla bean pods and orange slices. The result looks so beautiful and tastes even more delicious in elegant glasses.

I'll make him a fresh juice with watermelon and immortelle.

I'm going to make a green salad with spring dandelion greens, chive heads, and nasturtiums along with a salad dressing with olive oil, apple cider vinegar, raw honey, garlic, and a drop of thyme essential oil; it looks so inviting and fresh.

For the main course, I'll serve roasted sweet potatoes with herbed aroma butter and edible flowers on top. I'm also making thyme and sage-infused spring asparagus on the barbecue. Additionally, I'll serve tarragon, miso, and seaweed brown rice and perhaps something a little meaty for my man.

I made a rich chocolate mousse with vanilla, cardamom, and rose petals. That man just can't resist cardamom in any form.

It's a special night so I'm chilling high-quality French champagne with just enough rose syrup to flavor and flirt.

Once we've finished dinner and champagne, the real fun begins. I'll get him to take off his shoes and will lovingly wash his feet with warm water bathed with pine cone, white cedar, and cypress essential oils. I love a man who smells of forests and sweat.

I'll slowly tie a cashmere blindfold on him and introduce him to a variety of oils to awaken his nose and pump up his drive. I'll feed him honey laced with immortelle and cape chamomile and change it to cardamom and cinnamon. The warming action of those oils intensifies the whole evening. They go to all the right places with precision and speed. I'll massage his hands deeply and allow him to massage mine.

I'll bring him to my bed, turn the lights down low and light a stick of homemade incense and some beeswax candles. Oh the excitement. And then . . . well diary, some things are just too private for even you.

In anticipation of things to come,

Elana

aromatherapy for sensual living   *the scented diary*

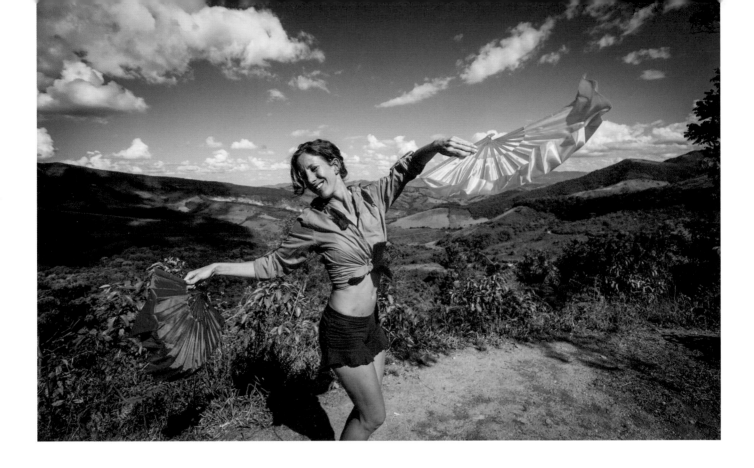

Sensual Living Manifesto

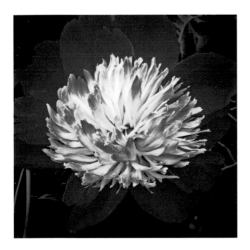

Here's to flower kissers, life lovers, tree huggers, meditation sitters, yoga flexers, ceremony seekers, mushroom pickers, leaf smokers, ecstatic dancers, super food munchers, and rainbow riders. I bow to you on your path to oneness. The divine expresses itself through you and, darling, you're beautiful.

I call forth all you beautiful bliss seekers to build a battalion of positive souls ready to beam their golden light into the world. We know that light eclipses the dark and we have infinite power to shine. In firmness, we spread our heartfelt iridescent love for all who are open to receive.

How do we do it?

1. Love is the answer.

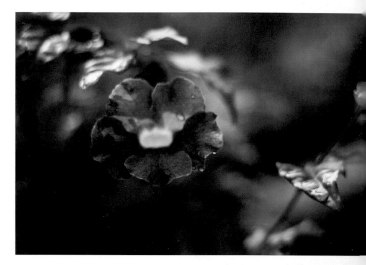

Love it all. Love is all we need. Love is all there is. Love heals the deepest fractures. Love softens the hardest stone. Love is without judgment or possession. Offer unconditional love to those in need for them to use as necessary. It could be a person, an animal, or the planet as a whole. It's the single best tool I have to move through the sticky points of life.

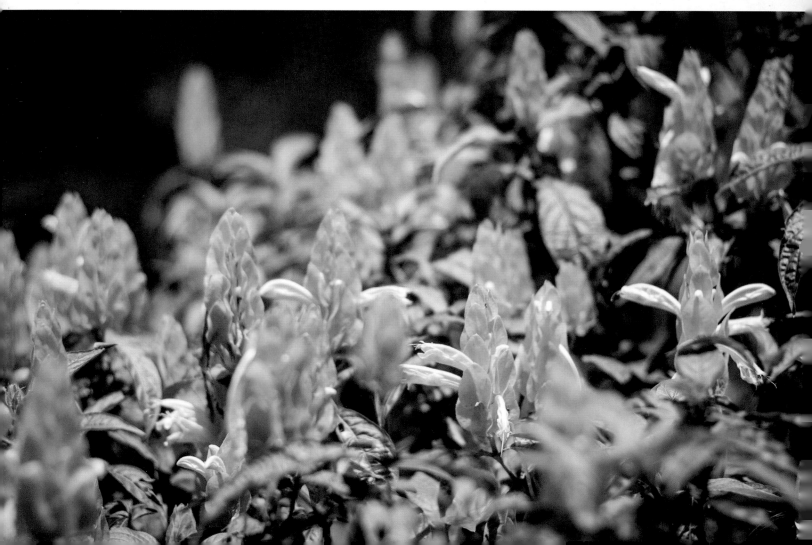

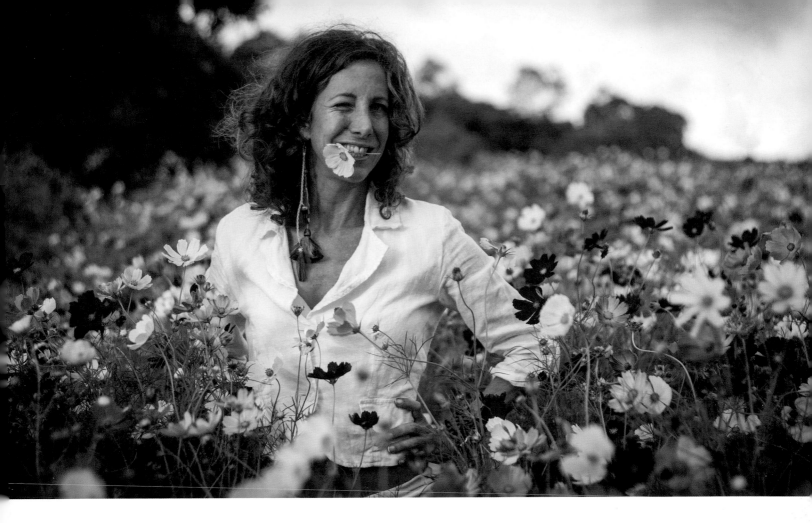

Allow the universal love vibration (God, Christ consciousness, Buddha nature, Allah, spirit, nature, energy) to enter and permeate your whole being. Succumb to it as you would a lover. Breathe it in and let it move into the tiny caverns of your lungs. Let it enter into your bloodstream and saturate your organs. Let it swim up your spine. Breathe in loving gratitude. Let it circulate in and out of your heart for the world to be inspired by it.

2.　Let nature take your breath away every day.

From splendidly colorful feathers to ascendant, intoxicating perfumes and majestic, breathtaking views, nature is begging for you to feast on her beauty. As you do, you'll become more inspired, peaceful, trusting, and whole. Commit every day to inhaling the miracle of life unfolding before your eyes. Witness the miracles outside and you'll very soon begin to see miracles happening on the inside.

3.   Practice health.

Our body is our temple. Nourish it with whole, vibrant foods and let it sing. Move it freely and regularly to feel confident, sexy, and engaged with life. Strength is sexy. Health isn't all that complicated. Most health issues can be solved with a smile, a glass of water, an apple, and a pair of sneakers. Gratitude is the quickest path to sublime ecstasy.

4.   Flirt.

Let life force energy ripple through your body to transform you into the luscious, coconut-scented exotic treasure that you are. Flirting doesn't necessarily mean lewd intentions. For me, flirting is an opportunity to connect, warm, and invite love to all whom I meet. I flirt with anyone with a glint in their eye and a bounce in their step. Old men, children, the cashier at the health food store. . . I try to sparkle a little sunshine dust for my benefit and theirs. Remember that a well-timed wink will take you places.

5.   When feeling stuck, make nature mandalas.

Go outside. Nature medicine is everywhere. It could in the forest, by the beach, or even in a small alleyway littered with weeds and wildflowers. Designate a quiet area to create your nature mandala. Let nature work through you. Collect items from your immediate surroundings such as flowers, twigs, feathers, leaves, grasses, acorns, bones, and rocks. Arrange them in shapes, patterns, or in whatever way spirit is calling you to create.

There's something enlivening about using nature as a canvas and touching living things to create art. Go back to it a few days later to see if the piece has changed or if spirit left you a gift.

6.   Be teachable.

Nature is gently, lovingly guiding us to be our best. Use the signs and symbols you see in nature as teachers to help you on your path. I look to animals, weather patterns, or repeated symbols that pop up in my life as thematic energies I need to pay attention to in order to correct myself if necessary.

If you approach your life with the eyes of a child and a willingness to learn, you will never get stuck in your ways or get old. You will be able to grow and develop to become the fully formed being you were intended to be. It's an opportunity to sip from the fountain of youth with glee.

7.   Invest in beauty.

I've been known to love champagne, cashmere, and sparkles. Beauty can be luxurious indulgence or simply tucking a flower behind your ear. Make beauty an important everyday directive. The more you invest in beauty, the more beautiful you'll be. It is the laws of attraction in action and you have all the power. Aim to include essential oils every day to remind you of the beauty that is ours to hold.

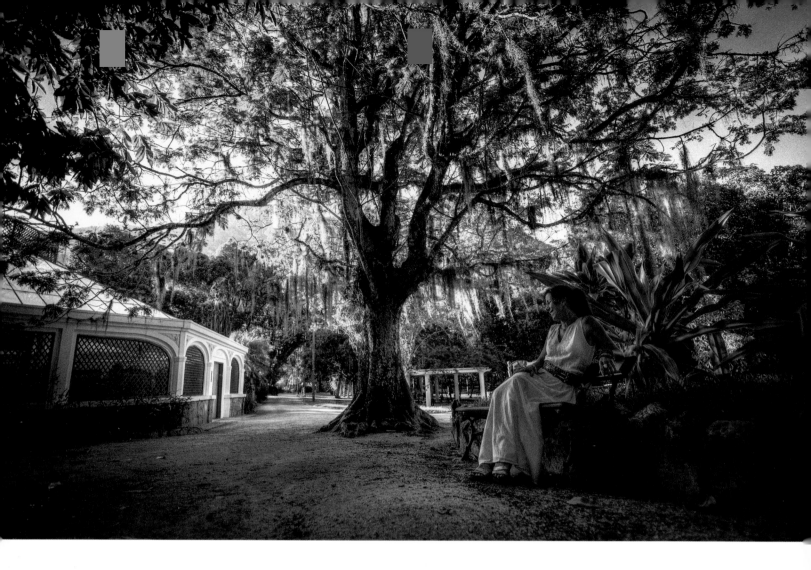

Essential Oil Personality Profiles

Each essential oil is a dear friend that I've known my entire adult life. In that time, oils have seen me through many personal incarnations, boyfriends, homes, careers, countries, both good and bad decisions. They've been with me every day in one or many different applications, without exception. The flowers never disappoint. I feel like I know them intimately and they know me too. When I want a big sister hug, I turn to lavender in the bath. When I want to feel like a sexual tsunami, I run jasmine through my hair. When I want to be bright, bouncy, and beautiful, I ingest tangerine.

When I'm in treatment with clients, I can smell a specific oil from inside the bottle and know exactly which one my client needs. It feels like the flowers are working along with me to help and heal. It's quite magical.

In each essential oil personality profile, you'll find a brief understanding of its uses, a description of its personality and its complementary oils. There are some that have more than one personality but, for clarity, this is a great place to start to familiarize yourself and develop your own relationship with them. The more you work with them, the more they reveal their secrets to you. I dare you to find new and innovative ways to incorporate them into your life.

Essential oils tell their intimate stories and have shown me their souls. I feel honored to speak on their behalf.

Bergamot

A springy Italian sprite with a sparkling smile.

Bergamot is a variety of pear-shaped orange found in Italy and traditionally used to flavor Earl Grey tea and confections like Turkish delight. While the fruit is bitter and inedible, the skin of the fruit provides a fabulous, effervescent essential oil that is powerful beyond measure. I use bergamot in my clinical practice to treat those who are negative, angry, and need a sunshine-filled boost of joy. Bergamot is a guaranteed happy-maker. It's a citrus oil, so avoid using it directly on the skin while in the sun as it will cause burns. Bergamot has a tangy, sweet smell that moves difficult and sticky emotions.

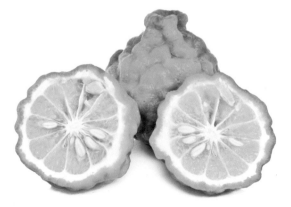

Bergamot is true bubbling positivity. He meets every day with enthusiasm and values the present moment. Bergamot is a solid friend. You can call him at any time of day or night and he will consistently, effortlessly show up to your needs. He is so happy and energetic that it's virtually impossible to stay grumpy when he is around. His smiles are deliciously infectious.

Bergamot is a tall, slender man with deep blue eyes and a smile that reaches from ear to ear. He is known to love ass-shaking house music and the simple pleasures of life. He is a beautiful soul with a kind heart and deep wisdom.

Bergamot is confident. He is a team player who works beautifully with lavender, ginger, tangerine, cinnamon, grapefruit, French cedar, fennel, and geranium. Bergamot is beautiful on honey or citrus-flavored desserts.

Bergamot is a sunshine-filled beam of happiness who is always on your side.

Black *Pepper*

A warm rebellious spirit

Black pepper is one of the oldest spices and was used as currency on the spice route during Attila the Hun's reign. It was found in the nostrils of mummified bodies and thus thought to be part of the mummification process.

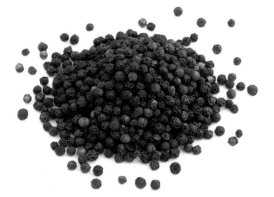

Black pepper is semi-toxic, meaning that sensitive people can have skin or respiratory reactions when they use it. But there is an advantage to being semi-toxic. It can efficiently move toxic and stagnant sludge out of the body. It's excellent for warming tight muscles, and dispelling gas and nausea. It can gently bring down a fever and is a potent aphrodisiac, especially for men. Black pepper has a rich and velvety aroma that enchants and tempts.

Black pepper is a misdirected bad boy who has a sweet spot for bookish girls in cashmere sweaters who smell like vanilla and tangerine. Too much of a good thing is a bad thing when it comes to him. He starts out soft but can aggravate in larger doses. He's warming, spicy, sensual, and gives great neck and shoulder massages.

He mellows out when jasmine, lavender, sandalwood, marjoram, or tangerine are around. He also likes the company of cardamom, tobacco, laurel, and hay. Don't judge black pepper for his unruly behavior. He just doesn't understand his strength.

Black pepper warms the heart and inner recesses of the body.

Black *Spruce*

Wildman of the woods.

Black spruce doesn't have the dripping sensuality or wide aromatic profile of other oils, but it has a precision and cleanliness that make it a sensational ally in many medicinal circumstances. Black spruce is excellent for treating any lung-related issue. When using it, you feel as though you're deep in the forest and able to take full cleansing breaths. Black spruce is also a wonderful brain tonic. I regularly add it to my bath soap to help clean out the morning fog and jump exuberantly into my day. It stabilizes the nervous system and helps tone and boosts the adrenals. It's like having a resplendent forest in your back pocket.

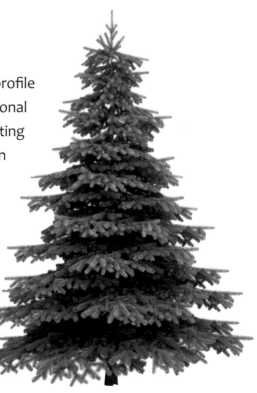

Black spruce is an elder. He's tall like a mountain with dark raven hair and wise and experienced eyes. He's loyal, authentic, and direct. Black spruce hails from deep within the Canadian forest where the life force is strong and the trees are enormous. This is what you get when you work with him: an overwhelming feeling of power, purpose, and poise. His love is deep but not mushy.

Black spruce is totally capable all on his own, but, like any good leader, knows the value of working within a team. He absolutely loves lemon, lavender, white cedar, vetiver, marjoram, palo santo, and sage.

Black spruce is a pointed arrow piercing through the heart of darkness.

aromatherapy for sensual living *essential oil personality profiles*

Cacao

The bliss of now.

Cacao is familiar yet exotic and hails from Ecuador, Brazil, Peru, Hawaii, Costa Rica, and many parts of Africa.

Most people have positive associations with chocolate, and for good reason. It's swoon-worthy-delicious and releases bliss molecules like serotonin in the brain. One of the more unique neurotransmitters released by chocolate is phenylethylamine. This so-called "chocolate amphetamine" causes changes in blood pressure and blood sugar levels, leading to feelings of excitement and alertness. It works like amphetamines to increase mood and decrease depression, but doesn't result in the same tolerance or addiction. Phenylethylamine is also called the "love drug" because it causes your pulse rate to quicken, resulting in that dreamy feeling of falling in love. It's full of bewitching and ecstatic delights for the mind, body, and spirit.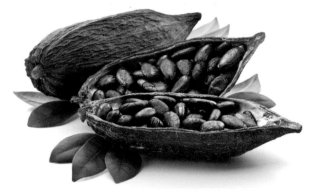

Cacao is deep, dark, delicious, intense, and powerful. With macho confidence, he'll touch you in all the right places to get your hips undulating to rhythmic beats. He'll hold your gaze and leave you breathless, spinning, and wanting more. He's so confident that he happily flirts with both men and women. Everybody wants a taste of his jungle juice. He can also be a little dangerous, which is part of his appeal. Too much cacao will make your head pound, your heart race, and leave you feeling woozy. Just the right amount will give you a post-orgasmic glow that lasts for hours.

Cacao always had a soft spot for vanilla. She'll always be his number one girl, though he can also charm lemon, cinnamon, ylang ylang, tangerine, peppermint, ginger, tarragon, fenugreek, and cardamom in a variety of ways and combinations. Cacao turns up the spice in every situation.

Despite being delicious, most cacao generally isn't suitable for consumption. Many distillations are from absolute extraction, so this one is better off left to massage oils, love butters, and perfumes. It's excellent for an after-sun treatment because of its high antioxidant content and ability to deepen a tan. You'll have a sun-kissed glow that lasts for days, and healthy skin to boot.

Cacao is a creamy, dreamy, decadent fantasy come to life.

Cape *Chamomile*

Beguiling but not so innocent.

Cape chamomile has a strong azure color and is traditionally used for calming a restless nervous system; improving sleep; healing blemishes, cold sores, and wrinkles; and acting as a strong anti-inflammatory. However, when combined with other oils, cape chamomile has an entirely different and sultry persona. It takes the form of liquid blue desire drops that bring in the divine to sacred sexuality.

Cape chamomile is a delicate young woman with soft, beautiful features. She's rather coy and enigmatic. When people are around her, they feel curiously peaceful and somewhat introspective. She causes them to pause. However, that is just one side of her personality. When you get her home with her man, she really comes to life. She's deeply sensual and most comfortable naked in the wilds of love. She's a surprise in the very best possible way.

Cape chamomile can be blended with immortelle, black pepper, cardamom, or frankincense to create an entirely flirty combination. Use it with sandalwood, geranium, lavender, frankincense, and neroli for skin care.

Cape chamomile is a sweet, pure angel and a sultry devil.

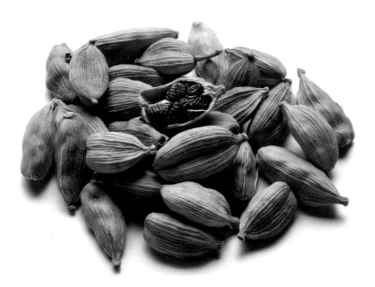

Cardamom

Wonderfully warming in all the right ways

Cardamom is one of my favorite oils. It has been used in ancient Greece, Egypt, and Persia for spicing dishes and in Arabic coffee. In the Ayurvedic tradition, it's excellent for expectorating phlegm. It's also used for treating digestive issues and healing urinary tract infections. Cardamom is wonderful at warming all parts of the body, especially reproductive organs, and is a potent, steamy aphrodisiac.

Cardamom is exotic and knows exactly how to tip her head at just the right angle to invite and entice. Cardamom is a major flirt. She slowly sways her hips on the dance floor with Eastern-inspired desi beats. She commands a potent power but is also deeply warming and immensely healing. She'll help you expectorate, calm your tummy, and give you a deep and loving hug.

Cardamom is a ravishing hottie to keep close to your heart and other parts.

Carnation

Sweet and spicy honeyed love.

Carnation flowers are used to connote love, admiration, fascination, good luck, and commitment. According to a Christian legend, carnations first appeared on Earth as Jesus carried the cross. The Virgin Mary shed tears at Jesus's plight and carnations sprang up from where her tears fell. Thus the pink carnation became the symbol of a mother's undying love and is the official flower of Mother's Day in

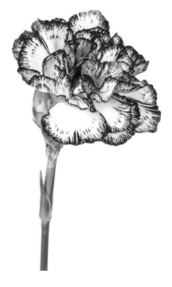

aromatherapy for sensual living *essential oil personality profiles*

North America. It's a favorite of writers and artists to help open the creative portal from where ideas and inspiration flow.

While I'm not in love with the flower, I absolutely swoon for the essential oil. It's, hands down, one of the most potent aphrodisiacs and is reserved for only the most special occasions. It decreases anxiety, warms frigidity, and is a key to open the door for magical nights. It's surprising that such a common flower has such an intoxicating and uncommon aroma.

Carnation can be described in one word: foxy. She's sweet and petite but, but for someone her size, takes up a lot of space. She's magnetic that way. She comes off as naïve but with a glint in her eye and a swagger in her step, it's clear that she knows precisely what she is doing. She loves indulgent luxury without apology.

Carnation is an unforgettable beauty who languidly lingers in the hearts and minds of those she touches. She's potent, so only use her in moderation. She's a lady who knows her worth and does everything with perfect precision.

Carnation is a euphoric, aphrodisiac, and base note. She blends beautifully with lemon, vanilla, lavender, rose absolute, hay, marjoram, and clove.

Carnation is a sexy siren whose scent will lift you up into the astral realms.

Cinnamon

Hot-blooded babe from head to toe.

Most people absolutely love cinnamon. It's used the world over in culinary and medicinal traditions. It's excellent for flavoring food or boosting the immune system. It clears pathogens from the stomach and has a wonderfully sweet and zesty taste. Cinnamon has been proven to be effective at balancing blood sugar levels in type 2 diabetes. I always add a drop of cinnamon to my morning smoothie for its favor and warming capabilities.

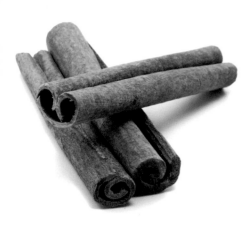

Cinnamon is one spicy number and can be quite a handful. She'll take over the dance floor and flirt shamelessly with every man there. With hips bumping and eyelashes flapping, she's pure heat and passion. You'll get burned if you don't handle her carefully, especially undiluted on sensitive skin. But at home, cinnamon is soft and nurturing. She'll rub your feet and whisper in your ears. She'll go deep into aching muscles and soothe them with ease. She'll knock any cold out of the body because of her fierce antibiotic and immune-boosting properties.

Cinnamon blends beautifully with cardamom, black pepper, vetiver, lemon, grapefruit, ylang ylang, sandalwood, tangerine, and vanilla.

Cinnamon is all class, sass and . . .

Clove

Mysteriously warming and curiously potent.

Clove is a fantastic medicinal oil used in many ancient cultures to treat tooth and gum infection, destroy parasites in the small and large intestine, and kick cold out of the body. It was first discovered in 1721 BC and has somewhat of a sordid history. The Dutch wanted a monopoly on cloves as they were worth more than gold, so they went about destroying clove trees that sprouted up anywhere outside of their empire. It was a native tradition in Moluccas (an archipelago within Indonesia) to plant a clove tree

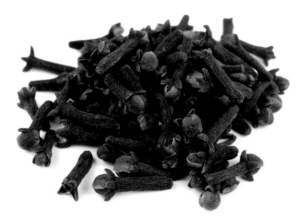

upon the birth of a child. The life of the tree was psychologically tied to that of the child. If something happened to the tree, it didn't bode well for the child it was associated with. Consequently, the Dutch weren't welcomed warmly.

aromatherapy for sensual living *essential oil personality profiles*

Clove is positively warming and a welcome addition to any immune-boosting blend. It can also be an erotic oil if used in small quantities and the right ways. Much like nutmeg, it can liquefy phlegm and help improve circulation throughout the whole body.

Clove is mysterious and doesn't crave attention like black pepper, ginger, or cinnamon. She's quiet in her power and almost dark in her ways. She sits at the back of the room cloaked in a woolly coat of dark ambers, oranges, and reds and observes everything with hawk-like eyes. She chooses her words carefully, as she's not one for frivolity or grandeur. Clove does her work with precision and grace and is a no-nonsense kind of gal.

Too much clove will certainly upset your tummy and make you sweat, but sometimes that's exactly what's needed. She knows what she's doing and is unapologetic in her power. She means business and doesn't mince words.

Clove is also known to help those with frigidity issues, and can be ever so effective in the bedroom. She helps to move stagnation and blood to areas that need it most and one drop is often all you need to light a fire inside. Clove and honey are one of the sweetest combinations for the mouth, belly or loins.

Clove blends beautifully with cinnamon, black pepper, cardamom, sandalwood, frankincense, ginger, vanilla, lemongrass, lime, lavender, tobacco, and vetiver.

Clove is a spicy combination of sex and candy.

Cypress

Clean, crisp, and utterly consistent.

Cypress is a deeply curative oil that can clear unwanted energies and stagnation faster than almost any other. Cypress is traditionally used in funeral processions to soothe the living and help the dead transition into heavenly realms. Despite having a morbid connection, this oil is anything but stale or heavy. It has a fresh and clear aroma harvested from the cypress evergreen tree found in many Mediterranean countries. Cypress is very effective in expelling phlegm from the lungs and reducing unwanted dimples associated with cellulite. It also helps with anxiety, cloudy thinking, depression, heartache, and sore throats.

Cypress is a strapping young fellow with broad quarterback shoulders, a warm and winning smile, and a booming tenor voice. He's consistently cool under pressure and is fabulous at helping sort out the frustrations and pains of those around him. He's an avid and accomplished rock climber and thrives in wide open spaces and sparklingly crisp mountain air. He knows how to lift moods, clear out emotional cupboards, and help all those in need.

Cypress works beautifully with lemongrass, white cedar, red cedar, juniper berry, lemon, black spruce, rosemary, basil, and sage.

Cypress is a blast of majestic mountain air.

Dill *weed*

Soft like a feather and swift like a bee.

Dill weed essential oil has a decidedly different aroma than the herb. It's softer, sweeter, and more etheric. Dill weed is a fantastic oil to help bring in breast milk and boost its nutritional quality. It's a superb digestive oil and is excellent for relaxation and circulation. In tea, through

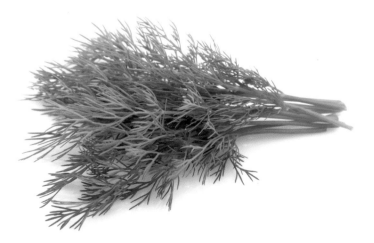

deep inhalation, or in the bath, it quickly takes the edge off and makes everything just a little more elated.

Dill weed blissfully floats on lily pads, taking in the glorious splendor of the day. She is sweet like a summer day and new love. With

aromatherapy for sensual living *essential oil personality profiles*

innocent and eager eyes, she's open to adventure and new experiences. Dill weed is heart-achingly beautiful and rock solid to the core.

Dill weed is easy, breezy, and gets on well with other culinary oils such as sage, rosemary, and thyme linalool as well as other fresh oils like cypress, lemon, juniper berry, and eucalyptus.

Dill weed is herbaceous champagne bubbles.

Douglas *Fir*

A breath of fresh air from way up there.

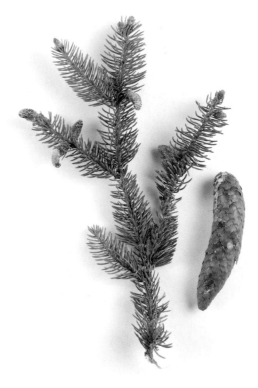

Douglas fir is a soft yet incredibly effective tree oil. It helps to open the lungs, clear the mind, and calm the nerves, and it's excellent for cleaning and treating wounds. It will lift the spirit and act as a powerful antidepressant. Douglas fir is one of the softer tree oils, which can be helpful for those with delicate lungs and constitutions.

Douglas fir is a sturdy lumberjack with a deep, bellowing laugh and a heart of pure gold. He's strong but surprisingly tender. For all of his gruffness, he's quite the lover. He takes his time because he knows that a woman's desire needs to be stoked and stirred, not set off like a firecracker. He'll open your lungs, free your heart, and get down on all fours to clean your floors. He'll steady your thoughts with his calm strength. Douglas fir will hold your hand in times of trouble, without even a quiver of uncertainty.

Douglas fir is good friends with white cedar, vetiver, lavender, geranium, marjoram, black spruce, sage, thyme linalool, grand fir, and lemon.

Douglas fir is a man's man and woman's wood-chucking fantasy.

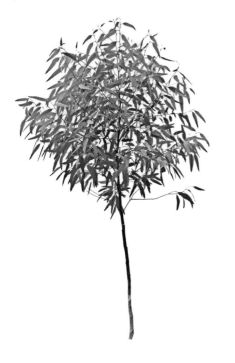

Eucalyptus

Multi-purpose aromatic medicinal.

Many people are familiar with eucalyptus as a way to combat an incoming cold or flu. It works quickly and efficiently to kill pathogens and keep you at your sparkling best. Eucalyptus leaf infusions containing eucalyptus essential oil were used by Aboriginal Australians as a way to combat body aches and pains, sinus congestion, fever, and colds. While most eucalyptus production has moved to China and California, the most prized oils still come from Australia. It's amazing for taming a throat infection, disinfecting countertops, and leaving your home feeling fresh and clean. Eucalyptus descends deep into congested lungs and sinuses and helps to efficiently clear breathing passages.

Eucalyptus is a compact warrior with beady eyes and energy to spare. He carries a sword and shield to battle any illness that comes his way. He's a little rough around the edges and speaks in guttural slang, but he gets the job done without wasting any time. He also has a degree of gentleness, though he can be shy to reveal that part of himself. He doesn't want other people to think that he's really just a softy at heart.

Eucalyptus is perfectly able on his own but — when combined with lavender, rosemary, or black spruce — he forms a dynamic superhero club of essential oil force. He has super-charged antibacterial power. When combined with tangerine, neroli, hay, or sandalwood, he simmers down and softens up to be a pleasant fresh-maker.

Eucalyptus is your go-to oil at the first tingle of sickness.

Fenugreek

A sweet innocent milkmaid fantasy.

Fenugreek is traditionally used in Indian food as a digestive aid and to increase milk production for breastfeeding mothers. It helps with inflamed skin and digestive distress, including constipation, diarrhea, flatulence, and nausea. Fenugreek is wonderful at helping to move stuck phlegm in the lungs and to ease bronchitis. It's sweet, deep, and smells somewhat like maple syrup. It's totally yummy and powerfully effective.

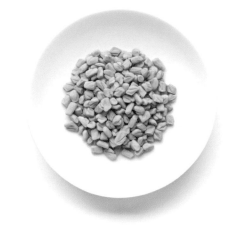

Fenugreek is a wholesome maiden with long, flowing blond hair that she often twirls into romantic styles. Her sparkling blue eyes invoke truth and kindness in everyone she meets. She has a special way of getting you to reveal all your secrets. Don't let her innocence fool you. In all of that sweetness and charm, she's also known to boost libido and get your juices flowing. She's an unexpected siren behind closed doors, but keeps that part of her personality hidden except for worthy suitors.

Fenugreek is good to have around if you're feeling blue because her sweetness overrides any sour situation. She gets on best with big sister immortelle and closest friend lavender, but also loves cape chamomile, sandalwood, grapefruit, and cardamom.

Fenugreek is your honeyed, perfumed petal friend with a scandalous wink you would never expect.

Frankincense

Soft-spoken ancient sage.

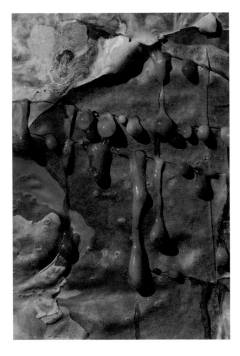

Frankincense is a magnificent aromatic resin that's been traded and, used for medicine, meditation, and a bit of magic for more than 5,000 years. It's often associated with the gifts given to baby Jesus, but that's just the start of the story. Frankincense is used cross-culturally to uplift and inspire, and is an excellent oil for meditation and spiritual connection. It's often used in church to invite religious communion and was burned in the streets during the plague. While people didn't know it at the time, burning the resin helped to purify the air from toxins stemming from the rotting corpses.

aromatherapy for sensual living *essential oil personality profiles*

Frankincense is outstanding in its ability to treat and heal wrinkles, scars, bruises, acne, and more. It's phenomenal for healing and fortifying the lungs and getting rid of a stubborn cough. In resin form, you can chew it to help reduce mouth and gum infections and support the entire immune system. It's also very effective at the time of birth for easy, harmonious labor.

Frankincense is a deep and handsome man with greying hair, strong hands, and a broad chest. He listens intently and only speaks when he has something important to say. His words are always exact, poignant, and full of love. You get the feeling that he's seen and done many things, but is utterly humble. He knows how to make you feel loved, cared for, and absolutely beautiful. He's a tender lover who will reach around and touch you in all the best places.

Frankincense is a rare gem with class and sophistication. He likes sandalwood, vetiver, lavender, tangerine, cypress, black pepper, immortelle, and rose absolute.

Frankincense is a conscientious lover with experience to share.

Geranium

Heart-healing flower power.

Geranium is often called the poor man's rose. While roses and geraniums are often grown together or distilled in co-distillations, geranium is anything but cheap. It has enormous healing and regenerative properties for emotions and the skin. It's slightly astringent, so it effectively opens and cleans skin

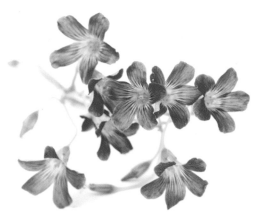

pores and is highly effective in any acne or mature skin formula.

Geranium is strong and mighty. She doesn't stand for sloppy and self-indulgent emotions. She'll go in, show you the truth of any situation, and clear mental confusion without apology. With loving force, she'll spank you back into your senses. Rose otto will do the same thing, but with silky, embroidered gloves. Geranium doesn't have the patience for that. She's a tall, broad woman with supple, glowing skin and an expansive and confident step. She stands straight and tall and, with one stern look, will encourage you to do the same. Geranium helps you stay on the righteous path.

Geranium is heroically strong and can easily rub out the delicateness of others in a blend, so use her sparingly or diluted. Geranium doesn't need others but knows that there's strength in numbers. She gels well with rose otto, rose absolute, lavender, marjoram, lemon, lemongrass, bergamot, spikenard, frankincense, magnolia, and tuberose.

Geranium is a dear older friend who has walked the road and knows many truths.

Ginger

A purring kitten who sits by the fire.

Ginger is used extensively in Asian and Indian cuisine for good reason. It's sweet, spicy, and a medicinal powerhouse. Ginger is excellent for nausea; stimulating the appetite; easing circulation issues; reducing inflammation; and supporting healthy liver function.

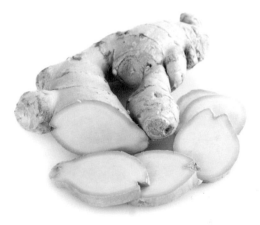

Ginger is everything you expect her to be: warming, a little spicy, and surprisingly strong. She lingers for hours, getting into the deepest parts of you without ever overstaying her welcome. She's a luscious redhead with ample breasts and womanly, wiggling hips. She wears a body-hugging scarlet dress that's a bit too revealing for her own good. But her warm heart and sweet laugh overwhelm any fashion faux pas.

Ginger is a social firecracker and helps party guests feel warm, comfortable, and grounded. She'll melt away any cool discomfort or stiffness in a room. Ginger is upfront, says it like it is, and never disappoints.

aromatherapy for sensual living   *essential oil personality profiles*

Don't be surprised if ginger gets you hot under the collar; she's a known aphrodisiac. By releasing sore muscles, healing tight and congested lungs, and calming nausea or an upset tummy, she gets blood flowing to all the right places.

Ginger plays well with other culinary oils such as cardamom, clove, cinnamon, lemon, grapefruit, bergamot, turmeric, and black pepper, and even likes to hang out with such exotic and erotic flowers as jasmine, carnation, and ylang ylang.

Ginger has a big, warm heart and a not-so-innocent wink.

Grapefruit

Insta-happy giggle juice.

Grapefruit is pure sunshine and good times; it has the amazing ability to lift the foulest mood with brilliant ease. Grapefruit essential oil moves sluggish circulation and works beautifully with cypress oil to remove stubborn cellulite. Grapefruit oil (in a small teaspoon of olive oil) boosts the productivity of the gall bladder and helps to break down congealed fats. It's highly effective in taming acne spots, but just be sure to use it at night since it's photosensitive and makes your skin more likely to burn in the sun.

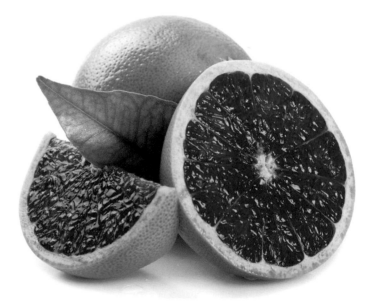

Grapefruit is a boisterous guy with a round, ruby face and an infectious laugh. He wears a loud Hawaiian shirt and exuberantly shakes your hand while patting you on the back just a little too affectionately. He'll offer you a tall glass of freshly squeezed citrus juice with a tiny colorful paper umbrella; he knows how to make you feel special. Grapefruit loves hosting parties in his opulent mansion overlooking the sea. While he has an effervescent personality, he also knows refinement. He collects rare heirloom fruit trees and super-charged healing crystals and happily shares his bounty with those he loves.

Grapefruit loves lavender, tangerine, bergamot, jasmine, sandalwood, cypress, neroli, tuberose, black pepper, cinnamon, clove, ginger, immortelle, and thyme linalool.

Grapefruit is a true blast of positivity and sparkling sunshine.

Hay

A sweet, happy girl with a Texas twang.

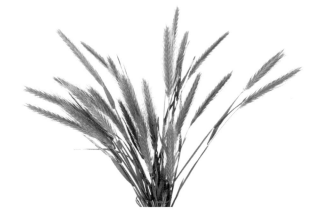

Hay (the grass that cows chew) is a relatively uncommon essential oil, but one of my favorites for blending. Hay makes everything fresh, light, and sweet. It goes beautifully in rich, heady, feminine blends and also works magic in masculine, earthy aromas. It pulls whatever it needs to harmonize a blend and make it sing. Many people think that they're allergic to hay, but more often it's the dust or mold that's contained in the plant. Pure hay essential oil smells like summer and youthful frivolity. It's a happy, sweet, and playful oil.

Hay is a beautiful girl with strawberry blond hair and sweet dimpled cheeks. She wears "Daisy Duke" cut-off jean shorts and a plaid shirt tied up way above her navel. She has an innocent and playful quality that can be surprising. She knows how to hang with boys and isn't afraid to get a little dirt under her fingers when invited to pitch in and help. She's able to easily lift any bad mood with just one drop of pearlescent sap.

Hay blends really well with lavender, black pepper, vanilla, Douglas fir, tangerine, neroli, sandalwood, cardamom, and clove.

Hay is boundless positivity and the living embodiment of long sun rays and endless summer days.

Keep her in your pocket and you'll always feel loved.

aromatherapy for sensual living *essential oil personality profiles*

Immortelle

The belle of the ball.

This essential oil goes by a few names, including Italian everlasting and helichrysum. It's a small yellow flower that grows easily in full sunlight. It's a powerful skin and cell regenerator that's extremely effective for bruises, wrinkles, burns, keloids, and stretch marks. Immortelle is fantastic for reducing liver and spleen congestion, and even helps with liver cell regeneration. My favorite way to use immortelle is as a sensual euphoric. The aroma is joyful, playful, and elegant and sends me right into a heart of a magical forest.

Immortelle is an opalescent forest queen whose intensity inspires poetry and potent lovemaking. She's dreamy, regal, and refined. In her long violet and periwinkle silk dress, Immortelle floats across the forest floor followed by fairies, divas, and elementals that humbly lay flower petals at her feet. You must listen carefully because immortelle, who tells grand stories of seduction and ascension, never shouts.

Immortelle is deeply feminine. She'll open you up to the most divine realms of consciousness and rapturous, pulsating pleasure. She is so elevating that it's almost narcotic. Mixed with other euphoric oils, she'll leave you intoxicated and floating on cloud nine, every time. She elevates your spirit and helps your soul soar into the god realm.

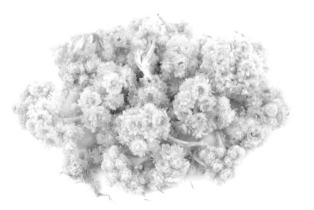

Immortelle blends beautifully with cape chamomile, rose otto, frankincense, lavender, sandalwood, cinnamon, laurel, and lemon. One of my favorite ways to tempt and tease is to use one drop of immortelle and one drop of cape chamomile on a half teaspoon of raw honey. Eat it slowly to experience waves of pleasure.

Immortelle delivers magical, all-knowing, and divine feminine power that leaves you quivering.

Jasmine

Hanky-panky petal perfume.

Jasmine is the undisputed queen of flowers with a refined elegance that works beautifully on everyone's skin. Jasmine picks up flowery, heady, and dewy notes on women and conjures musky and damp sexual flavors on men. It's called "moonshine in the garden" in India and ancient Indian paintings depicted lovers bathing in moonlight near jasmine plants. Jasmine is an aphrodisiac, mild sedative, and nervine tonic, and it's excellent for any female reproductive issue. It simultaneously tends to the heart and the loins, and is often obtained by absolute extraction so it can't be consumed.

Jasmine is unforgettable, exotic, and oozes expensive sophistication. She wears a flawless vintage 1920s white silk beaded dress that hangs stunningly on her subtle curves. Her thick, dark hair is tied up perfectly, with soft pieces caressing her gentle shoulders. You can't help but instantly fall in passionate love with her. She's beautiful and powerful inside and out. Jasmine is an erotic, euphoric base note with swagger to spare.

Just about everyone wants to mingle with jasmine. Who wouldn't want that rich and velvety aroma to exalt and elate them? Jasmine blends well with rose otto, tangerine, sandalwood, vanilla, tangerine, vetiver, lavender, lemon, black pepper, and cypress.

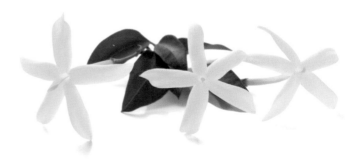

Jasmine is a delicious love story that you read between the sheets and never want to end.

aromatherapy for sensual living *essential oil personality profiles*

Juniper *Berry*

Super sharp shooter.

Juniper berries are used in the production of quality gin to produce its distinctive evergreen taste. Juniper is considered to be a sacred tree throughout the Himalayas and is burned in rituals and ceremonies because of its transformational effects. Juniper is similar to sage in that it clears and purifies unwanted energies.

Juniper berry is a powerful kidney tonic and my first line of defense when clients experience fatigue, kidney infection, or overall sluggishness. It's astounding at providing courage to face our deepest fears. Juniper berry has a fresh and clean scent that's both positive and effervescent.

Juniper is a chilled-out, easygoing guy who remains composed no matter what's thrown at him. When he arrives, people perk up, take a deep and satisfying breath, and then easily exhale. It feels good to have him close by because he's reminiscent of splendors of the forest and the enlivening effect nature has on our minds, bodies, and spirits.

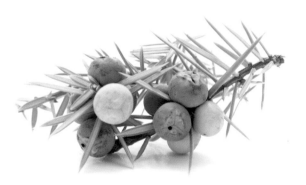

Juniper berry blends really well with other vitalizing oils such as cypress, lemongrass, lemon, rosemary, and black spruce. He's also loved by lavender, grapefruit, tangerine, sage, and thyme linalool.

Juniper berry is a brisk walk in the woods on an autumn day.

Laurel

All-knowing, multi-dimensional oracle.

Laurel has a fascinating history. In ancient Greece, wearing a laurel wreath indicated that you held the highest status and wealth. Laurel has also long been attributed to channeling divine energy. It was used to roof the temple of Delphi, which housed the Greek god Apollo's infamous oracle. Laurel has some witchy powers. I've used laurel to increase psychic abilities, clear the lungs, and sharpen the mind. Laurel is particularly effective at increasing dream states and bringing in prophetic dreams. It's also excellent for treating circulatory issues, cellulite, and edema as well as for boosting immunity.

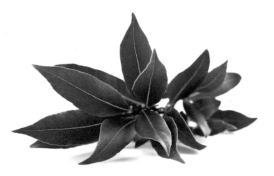

Laurel is a wild and strong woman with long and wavy hair that blows dramatically in the wind. She has piercing blue eyes that reach deep into your soul. One look and she knows all your secrets, past and present. Laurel is powerful, commanding, and deeply mysterious.

Laurel stands strong with her witchy sisters lavender, cape chamomile, and tansy, as well as medicinal brothers juniper berry, sage, rosemary, black spruce, and white fir. Laurel can be very kind and soft.

Laurel is a seductive mystery who illuminates only for the chosen.

Lavender

Lovely lady who's loved universally.

Lavender is the go-to miracle-maker. Lavender oil was used in ancient Persia, Greece, and Rome to clean hospitals and sick rooms and was highly prized by Roman soldiers who carried it in their first aid kits. Lavender is amazing for healing burns and pimples; easing female reproductive disorders; and alleviating mental/emotional issues such as anxiety, depression, and nervousness. It's outstandingly helpful in easing headaches, muscle aches, and exhaustion, as well as for repelling mosquitoes. It's also a reputed sleep aid.

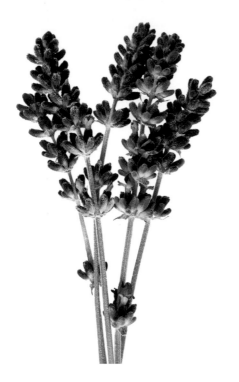

Lavender is the cheerful, smiling party host who tends effortlessly to her guests' needs. Some discount her ability because of her softness. That's an uncivilized miscalculation of her capabilities and wisdom. She consistently and lovingly delivers on her promises. She's a big sister who loves deeply and always has time for a hug, a chat, and some sound advice. She's incredibly kind, patient, loving and, of course, devastatingly beautiful.

Lavender methodically does her work with passion and quiet determination. She's humble, kind, and delighted to help wherever she can. She's both a devout holy sister and bubbly cheerleader, often in the same moment. Lavender can either elevate or calm any situation. She's such a good adapter.

Lavender blends well with just about everything. If you're working on a blend that's not forming properly, one drop of lavender will bring everything together in a cohesive package like a sparkling ribbon on top of a really beautiful box. Some of her closest friends are rose otto, lemon, blood orange, ylang ylang, vetiver, sandalwood, and bergamot.

Lavender is an all-around class act and a sparkling diamond.

Lemongrass

Get on the grass.

Lemongrass is a powerful, unusual oil. The aroma smells like pungent, exotic lemons that, interestingly, have nothing to do with citrus family. Lemongrass is a staple in Indonesian, Thai, and Vietnamese food. As an oil, it effectively and decisively works to eradicate stormy emotions, reduce pain and inflammation, bring down fevers (especially those associated with malaria and other tropical diseases), and is a fabulous antimicrobial and antibiotic. It's also a powerful insect repellent. When I was in the jungles of Peru, I was given lemongrass tea every morning to keep malaria mosquitos away. Thankfully, it worked. One of my favorite combinations is of lemongrass and ginger. It's surprisingly zingy and helps blood zoom all over the body. What a powerful pick-me-up! Lemongrass is an overall tonic that helps to clear the mind, support healthy digestion, and give users an invigorated calm.

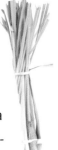

Lemongrass is an avid traveler who loves off-the-beaten-path Asian locales and syrupy umbrella drinks. Lemongrass is distinctive. He is handsome but not in a typical Hollywood way. His attractiveness comes from his rugged confidence and his unique way of seeing the world. He gives you a fresh perspective that causes you to reconsider everything you once knew.

Lemongrass can be somewhat overpowering in a blend so it is best to use him sparingly or on his own. He blends well with cypress, white cedar, lavender, ginger, lemon, clove, or cardamom.

Lemongrass is a freedom-loving leader with courage to spare

Marjoram

Peace, love, and happiness.

Marjoram is deeply relaxing and profoundly healing. It's particularly effective for those dealing with depression, anxiety, mood swings, or grief. It's a potent sedative and especially helpful for a tender-hearted soul going through a bad breakup.

Marjoram is a deep, bluesy woman who's whistling a song with a guitar strung around her neck. She's a true flower child whose very presence calms you down, helps you unwind, and enables you to fall into a very deep sleep. But for all of her chill, she's a wild child who doesn't bow to convention. She can be difficult and brash in a blend and can easily take over, though it's not her intention. She has a quiet, sweet, and caring disposition but can't control her strength.

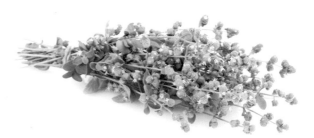

Marjoram likes to hang out with those who are also into chilling, like lavender, cape chamomile, geranium, laurel, vanilla, spikenard, and sandalwood.

Marjoram is a star child who is at ease in her own skin.

Neroli

Heaven on a Sunday.

Neroli is the orange blossom flower that blooms for two weeks in Mediterranean climates. It must be picked by hand and processed on site so as to not lose any volatile oils. It's hypnotic, ethereal, and euphoric. Neroli is particularly compelling in moments of expanded bliss with your beloved. It is one of my all-time favorite oils.

At the end of the Crusades, orange blossoms were woven into a bride's bouquet to ensure a hundred years of good luck, happiness, and fertility. A bride who wore orange blossoms in her hair was proclaiming her virginity. Meanwhile, in Madrid, ladies of the night wore neroli as a perfume to seduce and lure clients. As such, neroli symbolizes both seduction and sexual purity.

Neroli is effective at calming the central nervous system, making it an excellent antidote for insomnia. It's astonishing at healing scars, stretch marks, pimples, wrinkles, and dry, irritated skin. I add one drop of neroli to my laundry soap to aromatize my clothes. It's simply delicious.

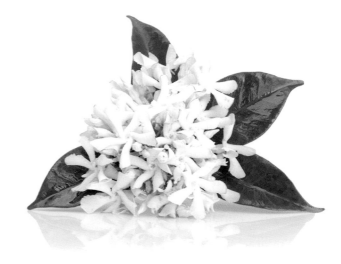

Neroli is a sweet and nubile maiden who luxuriates in vast flower fields. On her cream-colored blanket, she demurely eats tangerine-scented crème brûlée while sweetly singing "love is all there is." She has a playful, erotic, and captivating innocence to her. All those who see her fall instantly and unknowingly under her spell.

aromatherapy for sensual living *essential oil personality profiles*

Neroli prefers to play with those in her family (tangerine, lemon, blood orange, petitgrain, and grapefruit) or those that are equally refined and elegant, like jasmine, sandalwood, lavender, rose otto, and immortelle.

Neroli is a dreamy delight that, once smelled, is never forgotten.

Nutmeg

A delightful and insightful mind-altering trip.

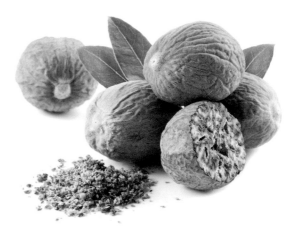

Nutmeg has a reputation for imparting a hallucinatory effect when smoked or consumed in large quantities, but that's not its whole story. Nutmeg is a tremendously powerful full body tonic. It helps circulate blood, dispel gas from the stomach and intestines and, much like clove, is effective in treating mouth and tooth-related issues.

Nutmeg has a compelling history. It was popular in ancient Greece and Rome as an effective brain tonic despite its high cost and rarity. The Dutch gave the British the island of Manhattan in exchange for nutmeg and sugar in South America. It's a powerful aphrodisiac because it warms all parts of the body and has a connection to confection and Christmas, which provides positive memories for most people.

Nutmeg is a dear friend with palpable warmth that emanates straight from her heart. She's a woman of diverse abilities and talents. She knows precisely what to do and say in every situation with elegant grace. She's contained and firm and, in the same moment, loving and soft. Nutmeg has an amazing ability to hypnotize pain so that it disappears out of mind and body. She can be surprisingly saucy and will wink at you in unexpected moments to expertly light sexy fires in your stomach and loins.

Nutmeg knows how to warm up a crowd and get it moving. She likes to hang out with other hotties like black pepper, cinnamon, and ginger for a deep muscle rub. She loves to cook in the kitchen with other culinaries such as tangerine, lemon, manuka, rose otto, and clove. She also flirts with cardamom, vanilla, ylang ylang, and thyme linalool.

Nutmeg is a nuzzling lover who shines pure light.

Osmanthus

Apricot, aromatic creamy dream.

Osmanthus is an erotic base note and a powerhouse of dripping sensuality. The ornamental orange-colored flowers are used in perfumery and blended with black teas to create full-bodied blends. The aroma starts off like plums bursting with juice and then fades to the smell of the well-worn leather of your favorite armchair, with hints of cherry, honey, and cream. Osmanthus is a costly erotic oil but well worth the price. One whiff will make you swoon and ache for more. It can easily be used on its own, as it has a complex scent profile that begs you to go deeper upon each inhalation. It's a one-way ticket to bliss on a jeweled magic carpet. It's opulent and quite heady.

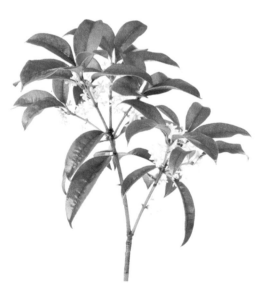

Osmanthus is a woman of commanding strength and beauty. She wears a deep red lipstick and has magnetic and distinctive charms. One look from her could bring any man to his knees, aching for more. She adorns herself with only the finest the world has to offer. Some might say she's snooty, but this queen prefers the term discerning.

Osmanthus has only a few favorites because she can take over and diminish the beauty of others in a blend. She mingles well with tangerine, vanilla, lavender, tobacco, and spikenard for evocative excitement. She's not one to share the spotlight since she shines brilliantly on her own.

Osmanthus is derived from an absolute extraction so only use it in perfumery or to scent your clothing — like on a blindfold, perhaps?

Osmanthus is succulent liquid charm.

Palo *Santo*

Wise humble healer.

While technically not a euphoric or an erotic, palo santo is definitely an exotic. It's a holy wood from the Amazon that's used in shamanic ceremonies to clear unwanted or negative energies. By burning the wood or inhaling the essential oil, you'll feel lighter, clearer, and more at peace. In oil form, palo santo has a rich and velvety aroma that mysteriously changes from black pepper to fir trees to butterscotch. It's an enigmatic shape-shifter like no other.

Palo santo is an old wizard with a long, flowing beard and a worn-out brown coat. He's a kind papa who will place you on his knee, dry your tears, and explain the nature of the universe in a clear, patient, and loving way. He digs into his pocket and pulls out the most amazing crystals, carvings, emblems, and amulets. He'll clear stagnation and foggy thinking from the third eye. He'll open and calm the lungs, relax an anxious mind, and aid in meditation. He's also known to help with inflammatory issues with ease and speed.

Palo santo is confident on his own, though he likes the precision of pine cone and all tree oils. He also works well with sandalwood, frank- 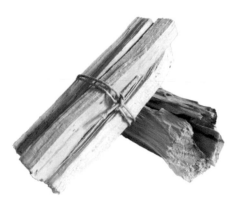 incense, citrus oils, patchouli, and vetiver. One of my favorite blends is called "the three teachers," which contains palo santo, sage, and tobacco. It's extremely powerful in moving out bad juju and replacing it with authentically positive vibrations.

Palo santo is a deep, magical, and mysterious.

Patchouli

Definitely not a dirty smelling hippie.

Patchouli, for many people, has a bad reputation. Synthetic, fractionated, or cheap versions have been overused as aroma bombs to combat the smell of reefer, sex, and absentee hygiene. Patchouli is anything but dirty. It's earthy, warm, smoky, grounding, and deep. It's a decidedly masculine oil that comes in different varieties from around the world.

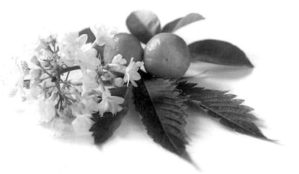

Patchouli has a rich history. Silk traders from China traveling to the Middle East during the eighteenth and nineteenth centuries packed their silk cloth with dried patchouli leaves to prevent moths from laying eggs because it's a potent insect repellent. Egypt's King Tut arranged to have ten gallons of patchouli oil buried with him in his tomb, as he was concerned that it might not be available in his afterlife.

Patchouli has an astonishing medicinal profile. It's a powerful sedating base note that positively communes with vetiver and sandalwood. Patchouli also works wonderfully for meditation and to treat sore muscles. It's very effective in helping to ease dandruff, eczema, and psoriasis. It's an effective deodorant and a subtle yet powerful aphrodisiac.

Patchouli is an intriguing, handsome man-god with curiously inviting eyes, strong hands, and a loving heart. He's an authentic spiritual Romeo who reads passages from The *Bhagavad Gita* and Rumi love poetry. He's a present, creative lover who attends to your every need for as long as you need. He leaves an impression so deep that, even when you recall him years later, you can instantly remember his touch, warmth, and sparkling smile.

Patchouli blends beautifully with sandalwood and vetiver to give base to any masculine and earthy blend. Patchouli also loves rose otto, neroli, lavender, marjoram, and black pepper for the ladies. He can glean a decidedly Eastern affection with cinnamon, cardamom, and spikenard.

Once smelled and never forgotten. Always pay for high quality oil.

Peppermint

Multi-faceted fresh-maker.

Many people have used or heard of peppermint essential oil because, like lavender, it's one of the most purposeful oils. Peppermint is outstanding for taming or helping avoid bug bites (especially blood-thirsty mosquitoes), calming a fever, easing an upset stomach, dispelling bad breath, combating foot fungus, lightening a foul mood, alleviating inflammation, and disinfecting wounds. The uses and benefits go on and on.

I've helped people in my clinic stop using asthma inhalers altogether with the use of peppermint. One drop in water is amazingly effective at internally cooling our bodies on the hottest summer days. Most people love peppermint because of its fresh and clean scent combined with its awesome medicinal power. It also tends to be less costly, making it widely available to anyone.

Peppermint is a stout little wrestler with energy to burn. He can easily pick and toss out just about any condition without breaking a sweat. He's precise in his movements and beloved by all. You can just about hear his fans cheering from the stands, *"Pepp-er-mint, Pepp-er-mint."* Our champion has a shaved head, bulging muscles, and the deepest blue eyes you've ever seen. He looks somewhat intimidating but, once he smiles, you know that he's nothing but sugar and spice and everything nice.

Peppermint tends to work on his own. He's so powerful that he often overwhelms those around him, but he teams well with tansy for inflammation and lavender to treat shock. He also likes rose otto, black spruce, cypress, and frankincense.

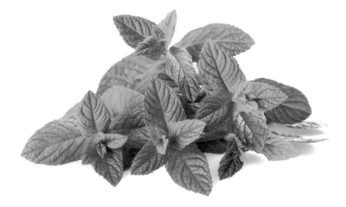

Peppermint is your on-the-go ice pack/first-aid kit in a bottle. Never leave home without it.

Petitgrain

A perky and positive caregiver.

Petitgrain is obtained from the twigs and leaves of the bitter orange tree but, unlike other citrus oils, it's not photosensitive. It's a true convalescence oil that helps restore health and vitality with ease and is excellent for calming the central nervous system and relaxing muscle spasms. It gently and lovingly guides you back to health with grace and speed as it's a powerful nervine tonic, skin regenerator, and all-over support for mind, body, and spirit.

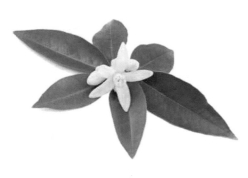

Petitgrain is a mild-mannered man who fits in everywhere he goes, and people unfailingly appreciate his presence. He loves singing James Taylor's "You've Got a Friend" and other 1970s soft rock classics. He's quiet and subtle in his energy, and never intrusive or overbearing like some of his friends. He lingers lovingly to support those who are going through a rough patch.

Petitgrain works beautifully with other citrus oils to enhance their potency. He also aligns well with geranium, lavender, and sandalwood to ease anxiety and stress. He likes cypress, juniper berry, eucalyptus, and tea tree for cleaning and restorative purposes.

Winter, spring, summer, or fall, all you have to do is call.

Rose *Absolute*

Late night, dimmed light woo.

Roses have a long tradition of being associated with love. Not surprisingly, all rose oils are extremely effective at treating and healing emotional heart issues. It takes sixty to ninety rose heads to produce one drop of rose oil, thus making it one of the most expensive, potent, and treasured oils in the aromatherapy apothecary.

Rose absolute is the wild and salacious cousin to the otherwise demure and delicate rose otto. She just can't be tamed; it's not her way. Rose absolute's behavior can be downright naughty but, because she's part of the rose family, she always maintains a degree of elegance and refinement. She's obtained by absolute extraction, which changes the aromatic and medicinal profile to one that's raw and lascivious.

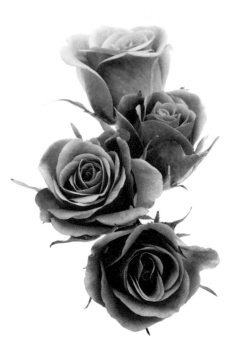

Rose absolute wears a black pencil skirt and a tight lacy red top with enough skin showing to tempt the imagination. She innocently bats her eyelashes to get whatever she wants, whenever she wants.

Rose absolute is a perfect perfume for attracting and netting your catch, but you simply can't swallow her whole (due to her method of extraction). She's incredibly effective at mopping up your tears and giving you a hug. She reminds you that fear is a pattern and love is a choice. She begs you to choose love.

Rose absolute is fiercely independent. She's loyal, loving, and pure once you get past her powerful sexuality. She blends beautifully with lemon, sandalwood, vetiver, geranium, grapefruit, lavender, vanilla, and tangerine.

Rose absolute is a big-hearted party girl who is out for a good time.

Rosemary

Spotlessly fresh.

Rosemary sharpens focus and concentration, clears away mental cobwebs, and even helps with hair growth. It's a powerful circulatory oil that helps release toxins, reduce cellulite, and boost low blood pressure. It's one of the most stimulating oils and is astounding at reducing arthritic conditions, inflammation, and overworked muscles. Rosemary is even being used in hospitals to combat superbugs that are simply too powerful for pharmaceutical drugs. Rosemary helps us come into the here and now. It also smells delicious on men's skin.

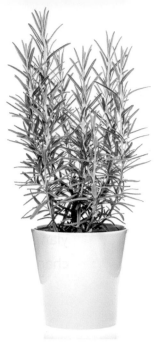

Rosemary is a go-getting type-A woman who is surprising in her strength. She's fastidiously hygienic and will clean your bathroom, disinfect your floors, and even clear your mind without any effort. She's focused and firm. She makes the complex simple and the disorganized neat. She's a no-nonsense, reliable straight shooter who is somewhat boxy and angular.

For all of rosemary's rigid strength, high standards, and expectations, she can soften around determined and resolute individuals. Some of her best friends are lemon, sage, cypress, palo santo, black spruce, oregano, thyme linalool, marjoram, tea tree, and eucalyptus.

Rosemary is a clear-headed Olympic swimmer who strives to do her best.

Rose *Otto*

The scent of love.

Rose otto is the steam-distilled rose essential oil and the most costly of the rose family. It's a powerful healer and regenerator for skin, wounds and wrinkles. It will soothe a sore throat and has unparalleled antibacterial properties. Rose otto tends to the heart and loins simultaneously. It's astounding at calming menstrual cramps, irregular periods, and warming a frigid soul.

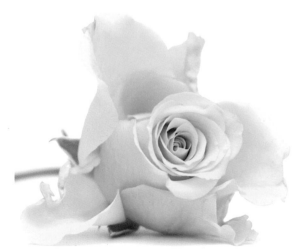

Jubilant roses are picked at the light of dawn and steam distilled so the oil can be eaten, adored, and adorned. Digesting rose otto is a magical, transformative, life-changing experience. Hearts open and love cascades. It's a sensation that's inward and outward, up and down. Rose otto makes the world a more kind and loving place to live.

aromatherapy for sensual living *essential oil personality profiles*

Rose otto is an elegant diva in a ruffled velvet dress who knows her power, presence, and poise. She's respected and revered by all of her peers as the almighty queen of flowers. She heals and loves with unwavering compassion. She's a best friend, mother, sister, and lover. The heart is our message center, as it connects us to the divine and navigates our lives. Rose otto is the global positioning system of emotional understanding. It's unparalleled in its ability to pacify emotional distress. She's an anchor, a lighthouse, and a loving hand when everything feels lost.

Rose otto is choosy as to who she hangs out with, but she really enjoys the company of ylang ylang, jasmine, lemon, tangerine, lavender, geranium, black pepper, cardamom, hay, immortelle, cape chamomile, and cardamom.

Rose otto will send you to the cosmos on a carpet of flowers with kisses on both cheeks.

Sage

Clean air and a clear mind.

Sage, like palo santo, is a remarkable plant used extensively in native traditions to remove unwanted or negative energies. It's done by burning the dried leaves and waving the smoke over a person or object to purify energy. It's a beautiful practice if you're feeling out of sorts. Sage, in Latin, is salvia — which means "to heal." And does it ever! The essential oil is a powerful digestive, has profound antifungal and antibacterial properties, and stimulates mental acuity.

Sage is an enigmatic character. It's difficult to describe him because he has the ability to alter his shape and features as necessary. He can be a curmudgeonly old man in one moment and a bold and brave hero in the next. The qualities that remain through the transformations are a commanding presence and a booming voice. You always know when sage is in the room. He tends to not be very social, but confesses his hopes and dreams to a few close friends.

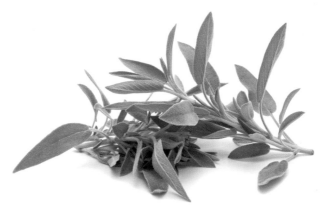

Sage loves the company of other clearing oils such as rosemary, white cedar, black spruce, cedar, palo santo, and tobacco. He also likes other herbs like thyme linalool, lavender, cypress, caraway, and spikenard.

Sage is a luminary with a formidable presence.

Sandalwood

My handsome heavenly prince.

Sandalwood is astonishing in its ability to restore skin's vitality and is especially helpful for dry, mature, and cracked skin. It's deeply grounding and excellent for meditation and aligning the chakras. In the Tantric tradition, lovers spread sandalwood on their bodies while celebrating the divinity of sexual ecstasy. Sandalwood, aloeswood, and cloves are the three incenses considered integral to Buddhist practice. Sandalwood smells wonderful on both men and women and is very safe and effective as a deodorant. It relieves depression and fatigue and is humble in its power.

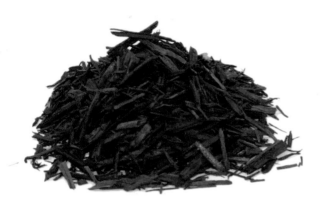

Sandalwood is wise, kind, and drips sophistication. He has years of experience under his belt and knows precisely how to charm the ladies. Luckily, he only uses his powers for good. He makes everyone feel their most beautiful, powerful and sexy. Sandalwood is suave and touches you with softness and quiet determination. His warmth slides deep inside you almost without you knowing and makes you ache for more. He'll heal your skin, mend your heart, and soothe your mind.

Sandalwood is a major flirt. He could hang out with just about everyone and get along with them famously. He especially loves rose otto, spikenard, frankincense, palo santo, grapefruit, cardamom, vanilla, and lavender.

Sandalwood is a dapper and dashing gentleman with serious woo.

Spikenard

Wise and loving grandmother.

Spikenard was the second essential oil I ever bought. Immediately upon smelling the amber-colored root oil, my heart opened to a deep love and ancient wisdom that I understood from a former lifetime. Spikenard has history.

Mary Magdalene used her mane to anoint Jesus' feet with spikenard at the Last Supper. At that time, the oil was a prized and costly perfume, more dear than gold. She was criticized by the disciples for using the oil on Jesus rather than selling it and giving the money to the poor. Jesus rebuked their criticism and told them to leave her to use it as she pleased. Spikenard is wonderful for anointing the soles of the feet and the top of the head to increase peace.

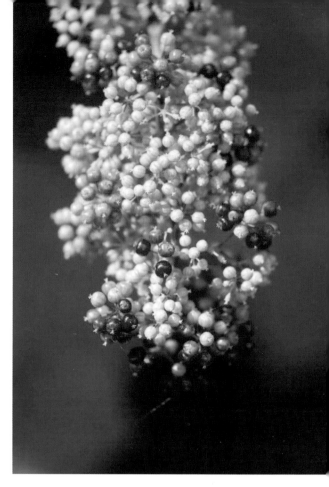

Spikenard is a benevolent sage with infinite patience and beatific kindness. She's a curvaceous and strong woman with thick greying hair braided down her back. She'll greet you after a long journey with a loving smile and a piping hot bowl of soup and crusty, buttered bread. By the roaring fire, she'll entertain you for hours with long and detailed stories of her adventurous life. Spikenard is excellent for relaxation, soothing a chaotic mind, and allowing harmonic resonance throughout the body. She'll alleviate inflamed joints, ease difficult menstrual symptoms, and love you unconditionally.

Spikenard loves her friends deeply. She treats them like her children and is particularly fond of lavender, lemon, cypress, sandalwood, hay, marjoram, palo santo, tobacco, and grapefruit.

Spikenard is a kind and generous soul who gives unconditionally from her heart.

Love is all there is.

aromatherapy for sensual living *essential oil personality profiles*

Tangerine

Blissful joy juice.

Tangerine makes everybody joyfully happy. Once consumed, it pushes positive rays of sunshine from the inside out in rainbow cascades of laughter and jubilance. Tangerine is excellent for treating any stagnation in the body, especially cellulite. It helps stimulate adrenals and reduces stress. Tangerine boosts moods and is very effective for treating postnatal and seasonal depression. Using tangerine in mop water makes for a cheery and clean home.

Tangerine is the good-natured, dimple-cheeked captain of the football team who is kind, loving, and surprisingly strong. He effortlessly boosts the whole team's spirit with a well-timed joke and his winning smile. Aside from being popular and positive, he encourages us to remember that life is beautiful and we're here to shine. He does the heavy emotional lifting and liquefies stagnation like a superhero. Nobody does it quite like tangerine.

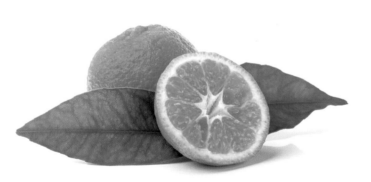

Tangerine loves hanging out with citrus oils, lavender, vanilla, cinnamon, palo santo, black pepper, fennel, immortelle, rose otto, frankincense, lemongrass, and nutmeg, and he can alter his shape and scent to help others come to their fullest light.

Tangerine is a loyal friend who always has your back.

Tarragon

Familiar yet curiously exotic.

Tarragon is an outstanding culinary herb and oil that was known in the Far East as the "little dragon." It has magical otherworldly properties and is extremely effective in three important ways: it helps secrete gastric juices; it improves circulation to every part of the body; and it acts as a mild stimulant. These properties make tarragon an unexpectedly powerful and erotic essential oil.

Tarragon is a true angel. His sweet lemony aroma floats up to the crystal kingdom where cherubs rest on clouds and sing lullabies in sweet harmonic resonance. Tarragon is a soft-spoken, incredibly intelligent young spirit who astutely absorbs information from all around him. He's amazingly contained for someone of his age and wise beyond his years. He has mystical powers and people seek his counsel in matters of the heart, stomach, loins, and mind. He has extraordinary solutions for anyone's woes but not for pregnant women.

Tarragon is a social guy. He likes to get out and mingle and, because of his magnitude, is able to satisfy many with only a small amount of energy. His most trusted allies are those that fulfill the same functions as he: culinary oils like rosemary, dill, oregano, sage, and thyme linalool; circulation oils like black pepper, cypress, juniper berry, and lemongrass; and erotic oils like fenugreek, jasmine, sandalwood, and neroli.

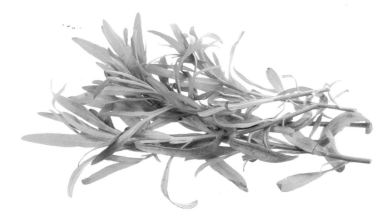

Tarragon is a euphoric delight with glints of gold.

Tea *Tree*

All hail the chief.

Tea tree is a well-known Australian antibacterial. It's amazingly effective at keeping infection at bay and cleaning out a wound. You can also clean your entire bathroom, including the toilet, with it. It's lovely to lift the lid to a pleasant aromatic surprise. Tea tree will tame pimples, kill athlete's foot, destroy head lice, and quash the fungus associated with yeast infections. (Dilute it if you're using it internally.) Tea tree is also effective at helping relieve the itch associated with insect bites. Tea tree oil was widely acclaimed as a near perfect antiseptic in the 1930s and 1940s and it was issued in Australian soldiers' first aid kits in the Second World War.

Tea tree is an army captain who gets the job done and doesn't tolerate any nonsense in his battalion. He has no time for flowery poetry or long and languid exchanges. There's a battle with bacteria and failure isn't an option. He's short on words and big on power. His hair is immaculately shaved while his pants and collared shirt are always perfectly pressed and starched. Tea tree destroys dirt, grit, and bacteria with ease and a hefty salute.

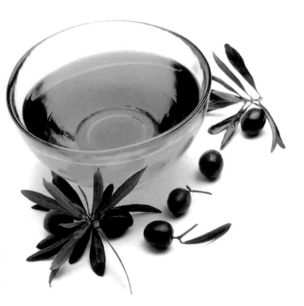

Tea tree will only tolerate others who have a strong work ethic and a commitment to getting the job done right the first time. He likes rosemary, black spruce, white fir, cypress, juniper berry, thyme, oregano, and lemon. I've seen rose otto flirt with him, too. She has a thing for men in uniform.

Tea tree is a panacea cure-all who just won't quit.

aromatherapy for sensual living *essential oil personality profiles*

Thyme

Herby little aromatic wonder.

Thyme was used in ancient Egypt as part of the embalming process, and ancient Greeks burned thyme sticks to cleanse the air of unwanted spirits and impart courage.

There are several varieties of thyme, though thyme linalool is my favorite. Unlike other thyme oils that can cause irritation or sensitivity, thyme linalool is kind and gentle to the skin and stomach. Thyme is highly prized for its ability to relieve gas, treat a vengeful pimple, or clear out mental mud. On men's skin, it smells like mojo-laced man sweat and honey. Thyme is often used in the kitchen to preserve meat and make it more digestible. The association with food and sex is palpable.

Thyme is unassuming, approachable, and an all-around wonderful guy. He's an activator and knows how to meet and mingle with many. His brown, messy hair can sometimes be a little unkempt but he's too busy to care. He'll pick you up off the ground and give you a bear hug and spin you around. He has exuberance and zeal to spare.

Thyme has many friends since he's so easygoing and flexible. He's a digestive powerhouse with sage, rosemary, lemon, and black pepper. He's a soft and sensual lover for men when combined with lavender, patchouli, lime, and black spruce. He's an effective room freshener with white cedar, lemon, and hay.

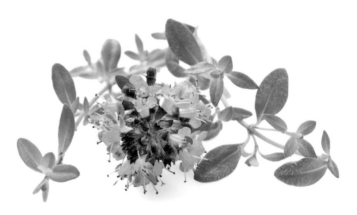

Thyme is a springy field of flowers beneath your feet.

Tobacco

A rough and tumble cowboy.

In native traditions, tobacco is a teacher plant that's used to call in ancestors, clear away emotional stagnation, and cure heartache. In some shamanic practices, medicine men are encouraged to smoke for forty days and then quit for forty days to work with the medicinal properties of tobacco without getting hooked. The Mayans offered tobacco smoke to the sky gods by blowing it toward the sun and the four points of the earth. It's powerful and divinely inspired stuff.

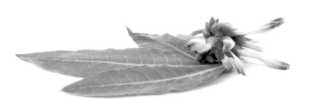

Tobacco in oil form is a hot and sexy lonesome cowboy who wears a ten-gallon hat, boot spurs, and well-worn chaps. He smells of leather and smoke and is weathered and wizened from his time on the road. Tobacco is the revered hero who saves the town, gets the girl, and rides off into the sunset without breaking a sweat. He has a sexy swagger and oozes masculine sensuality and confidence.

Tobacco loves to hang out with other masculine oils like palo santo, white fir, white cedar, cypress, sandalwood, vetiver, and patchouli. He also has a sweet spot for the ladies and gets down with jasmine, ylang ylang, marjoram, and neroli.

Tobacco is a sultry hottie who knows his game.

Tuberose

High-frequency passion poetry.

Tuberose is a night-blooming flower that's incredibly intoxicating, deeply sensual, and highly euphoric. It has a creamy, honey-like, spicy flavor that's similar to neroli, though more commanding. Throughout its flowering life cycle, tuberose changes its smell from camphor in the opening; a dewy, sweet mushroom and sex when in bloom; and slightly rotten meat when browning. It's a powerful, mind-altering aphrodisiac that's excellent for treating depression, anxiety, or any emotional issue. It's also a reputed anti-inflammatory oil and is used for deep grounding. It's used heavily in commercial perfumes because of its aroma and strength. Even one drop in twenty-five milliliters of carrier oils is strong enough to wear as a perfume for both men and women.

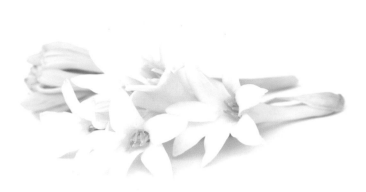

Tuberose is ancient in her knowledge and has so much to tell if you have the time. She'll send you to ancient mystical lands where beauty is revered and rejoiced. It's a leisurely place where people drink flower petal tea and ruminate on the flawlessness of the divine. Her pure white blossoms are euphoric, complex, and majestic. Tuberose will only reveal herself to those she deems worthy.

Tuberose stands elegantly on its own as a perfume but also blends beautifully with lemon, lavender, vetiver, palo santo, vanilla, fenugreek, lemon, tangerine, tarragon, and hay.

Tuberose is a true luxury for a chosen few.

Vanilla

Va-va-va-voom!

Vanilla isn't the bland, boring default of the food and flavor industry. It's bold, sexy, and warming, with just a little spice. Vanilla is an undisputed aphrodisiac and simply thrilling when anointed to lips, hips, or wrists. It's commonly used in perfumes because of its inviting, familiar smell. It works for both men and women as it mixes beautifully with different aromas and body temperatures. Vanilla is derived from the orchid plant from Madagascar and is obtained using

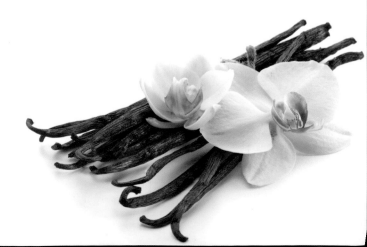

a CO_2 extraction, making it suitable for ingestion. Vanilla is powerful as a sedative and a stimulant. Additionally, it is mildly intoxicating and definitely provocative.

Vanilla is sophisticated, refined, and leaves a lasting impression. She prefers beeswax candles and fine French champagne. She wears a fitted cream Chanel suit with only the finest silk lingerie underneath. She's a lady in every possible way. She reveals herself slowly in a blend, lending her magic to others in order for them to come into their fullest expression. Her deep and warming properties are good for releasing sore muscles, aiding an upset tummy, and getting your engines roaring.

Vanilla blends well with tangerine, cardamom, fenugreek, cinnamon, ylang ylang, cape chamomile, vetiver, neroli, and bergamot. She also mixes beautifully with any of the warmer culinary oils and gives a blend a sweet and sultry flavor.

Vanilla is deep throbbing jungle magic.

Vetiver

Smoldering and smoky siren.

Vetiver is a delicious steam-distilled root that's effective for so many things, including being a mind-scrambling aphrodisiac. Vetiver is very effective at helping to ease anxiety and tension; it can calm even the most high-strung people. It's one of the most grounding base notes and is excellent for meditation

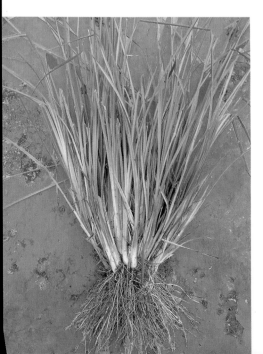

and auric cleansing. Its rich brown color and slow viscosity are invitations to go down and deep. I positively love the smell of vetiver on men's skin. It's lusty dripping alchemy at it's best.

Vetiver is mysterious and smoky in all the right ways. Energy descends from him into the darkest, deepest, and most enticing places. Vetiver is enigmatic and wraps himself around you like a brown cashmere blanket, hugging, squeezing, and tickling you with knowing aroma hands. Because vetiver is a root, he lingers languidly for hours, loving you intensely and slowly. He'll even call you the next day to thank you for your time together.

Vetiver blends beautifully with tobacco, white cedar, sandalwood, and patchouli for a deeply grounding men's cologne. It also mixes wonderfully in a massage oil with lavender, lemon, cypress, jasmine, laurel, and cinnamon. It will work anywhere you need to deepen and strengthen.

Vetiver is a classy gentleman with sway.

Ylang *Ylang*

Silky and sweet Oriental seductress.

Ylang ylang is sometimes called the cheap man's jasmine. That's an unfair title for such a beautiful, rich, and curative oil. Ylang ylang is deep and mysterious and stands alone as a powerful healer. It's known by several names, but it's from the Philippines' Tagalog language that the tree came to be known as ylang ylang — or, more correctly, álang álang, a term meaning "flower of flowers." It's wonderful for treating shock or emotional stress, reducing high blood pressure, and is a reputed aphrodisiac to treat impotence and frigidity.

Ylang ylang's deep richness blooms like a high-heeled lady strutting her stuff in a vintage gold and black Gucci dress in Tokyo's high-rent Ginza district. She'll find you on the street, grab you, kiss you passionately, and then run away giggling, leaving you breathless and baffled by the exchange. Ylang ylang is a powerhouse of dripping sensuality who won't take no for an answer. She's audacious and definitely not for everyone. Subtlety just isn't her thing.

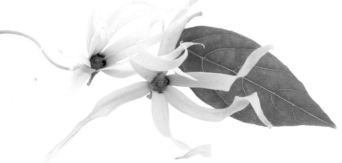

Ylang ylang blends beautifully with lavender, lemon, tangerine, ginger, black pepper, hay, clove, osmanthus, geranium, and sandalwood. She'll turn up the heat in any combination.

Ylang ylang will throw you down to scandalously smell the flowers.

aromatherapy for sensual living *essential oil personality profiles*

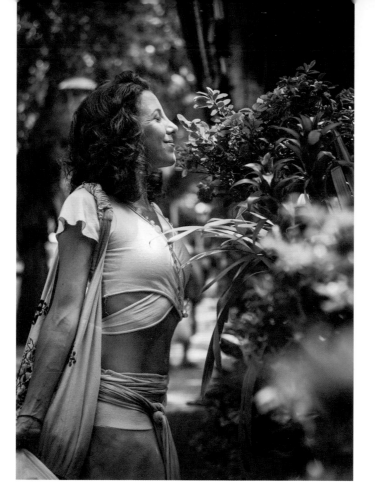

Classic Blends and Kits

Real *to the Feel Blends*

Clients are always asking me for easy, classic blends. Here are some of my all-time favorites. For these blends, use a ⅟₁₆ oz bottle topped with jojoba. You can easily scale the blend to a larger bottle in the correct concentration. There are roughly 100 drops in a ⅟₁₆ oz bottle.

In this concentration, I recommend these blends for perfume, air fresheners, and putting on sheets, clothing, hair, and more.

Simple Romantic

- three drops of rose otto
- three drops of sandalwood
- three drops of lavender
- one drop of tangerine

Racy Woman

- two drops of cinnamon
- two drops of cardamom
- one drop of vanilla
- three drops of tangerine
- one drop of jasmine

Racy Man

- two drops of sandalwood
- two drops of vetiver
- two drops of patchouli
- two drops of immortelle
- two drops of black pepper
- one drop of bergamot

Light and Bright

- three drops of grapefruit
- two drops of vanilla

- two drops of tangerine
- one drop of lavender
- two drops of cypress

Earth Magic Woman

- two drops of sandalwood
- two drops of hay
- two drops of lavender
- one drop of frankincense
- one drop of ylang ylang
- one drop of lime

Earth Magic Man

- two drops of white cedar
- one drop of patchouli
- two drops of sandalwood
- one drop of vetiver
- two drops of red cedar
- one drop of cypress
- one drop of juniper berry

Intuition Ascension

- one drops of cape chamomile
- one drop of tansy

aromatherapy for sensual living *classic blends and kits*

- one drop of geranium
- two drops of sandalwood
- two drops of lemon
- two drops of laurel

Wise Woman

- three drops of spikenard
- two drops of lavender
- two drops of immortelle
- two drops of sandalwood

Clear Mind

- two drops of cypress
- two drops of rosemary

- two drops of lemon
- one drop of lemongrass
- two drops of black spruce
- one drop of frankincense

The Teachers

- three drops of sage
- three drops of palo santo
- one drop of tobacco
- two drops of white cedar
- one drop of lavender

Kits

People often ask me what oils to buy if they're just starting out with aromatherapy. Here are different kits to help you delve into the world of aromatherapy with confidence:

First Aid (The Desert Island Kit)

Lavender, tea tree, peppermint, ginger, eucalyptus, oregano

Uses: respiratory conditions, colds, flus, burns, bruises, sprains, motion sickness, antibacterial, antifungal, antiviral, antiseptic, decongestant, expectorant, stimulant, bug bite prevention, fevers

Applications: inhalations, internal, bathing, compresses, suppositories, room spray, body spray, neat in certain cases (lavender with burns)

Erotic, Exotic, Euphoric Kit

Rose otto, immortelle, neroli, sandalwood, jasmine, cape chamomile

Uses: anywhere you want to include essential oils to make any experience more sensual

Applications: lovemaking, massage, internal (except jasmine), room spray, perfume, on sheets, bath, personal lube, meditation, heart healing, ascension

Culinary Kit

Tarragon, cardamom, rosemary, thyme, tangerine, cinnamon, ginger

Uses: in place of herbs, spices, or fruit to impart a full flavor experience into any dish you make, powerful antibacterial, and immune support

Applications: in food, smoothies, tea, honey, chocolate, salad dressing, soup, cookies, sorbet, herbed butters (all in moderation)

It's So Sexy Kit

Cinnamon, jasmine, vanilla, fenugreek, black pepper, immortelle

Uses: to tempt and tease a lover, invite the divine into the love space by aligning with the power of essential oils in the most intimate way; ignites sexual centers, potent aphrodisiac, improves circulation, relaxes mind and body, improves confidence, helps blood flow, supports being present, removes inhibitions

Applications: massage, room spray, perfume, on sheets, bath, personal lube (except black pepper), internal application on fruit or honey (except jasmine), tantric meditation

Trees Kit

Black spruce, red cedar, white fir, Douglas fir, French cedar, white pine, cypress, juniper berry

Uses: clears mind and lungs, improves circulation, assists meditation, powerful cleaning tool, strong antibacterial, treats exhaustion, reduces inflammation, expectorant, boosts kidneys and adrenals, sharpens senses, improves detoxification pathways, calms anxiety

Applications: cleans floors, air, toilet; inhalation, compresses, bathroom spray, on sheets, on vacuum bag, in laundry soap, sink, sauna, diffuser, lymph brush

Heart Healer Kit

Rose otto, geranium, lavender, spikenard, jasmine, marjoram

Uses: heals a broken heart, dispels shock, improves heart function, decreases apathy, depression, abandonment, insomnia, potent aphrodisiac, removes grief, powerful sedative, nervine tonic, excellent for wrinkles, herpes, shingles, mature skin, supports female reproductive system, anti-inflammatory, anti-stress

Applications: inhalation, bath, compresses, internal (except jasmine), anointed to heart and crown chakra, massage, room spray, on sheets, in hair

Deeply Grounding Kit

Vetiver, sandalwood, patchouli, frankincense, clove, osmanthus

Uses: sedative, relaxant, grounding, helps ease insomnia, mental/physical exhaustion, depression, general tonic, cell regenerator, eases aches and pains, cleans auric field, powerful meditation oils, aphrodisiac, calms anxiety, stress, good for mature skin

Applications: bath, inhalations, massage, anoint third eye and crown, room spray, perfume, on meditation pillow, in shoes to support grounding

The Middle Path Kit

Lavender, cypress, laurel, juniper berry, rosemary, lemongrass, fennel

Uses: antidepressant, antiseptic, treats headaches, mood swings, anger, general detoxifier, stimulates blood flow, bile production, reduces cellulite, improves mental clarity and concentration, fungicide, insecticide, minimizes aches and pains, brings body into alignment, strengthens connective tissue, general toner, anti-inflammatory

Applications: massage, bath, perfume, scrub, compresses, around floorboards or on skin to prevent insects, in laundry, on sheets, sauna, lymph brush

Uplifting Kit

Tangerine, petitgrain, grapefruit, hay, lemon, neroli

Uses: antiseptic, mood enhancer, stimulant, detoxifier, tonic, boosts digestion, improves mental clarity, improves concentration, detoxifying to kidneys and liver, powerful astringent, disinfectant, sauna, diffuser, reduces feelings of anger, promotes positive feelings

Applications: inhalation, internal, diffuser, room spray, in laundry soap, cleanser, bath, on sheets, in food

Note: Avoid use in direct sunlight, as photosensitivity may occur

Supreme Clean Kit

Thyme, black spruce, tea tree, rosemary, sage

Uses: powerful cleanser for internal and external applications, effectively rids insects, mold, bacteria, fungus, moths, strengthens mental acuity, clears lungs, unblocks the mind

Applications: mop floors, effectively cleans bathroom, wash and disinfect kitchen surfaces, room spray, pet wash, laundry soap, to combat fungus in feet, dropped inside stinky shoes, in garbage bin, used along floorboards to deter pests

Anti-inflammatory Kit

Turmeric, cypress, immortelle, lavender, rosemary, rose

Uses: calms and soothes inflammation inside and outside the body

Applications: compresses, salve, inhalation, massage, bath

Anti-stress/Relaxation Kit

Lavender, marjoram, cape chamomile, sandalwood, neroli

Uses: relieves stress, tension, anxiety, depression, frustration, grief, headaches, muscle tension, sedative, reduces bruises, pain, helps achieve a sense of deep inner peace

Applications: perfume, room spray, massage, inhalations, warm compresses, bath, sauna

Muscle Tension Kit

Black pepper, lavender, grapefruit, clove, peppermint

Uses: relieves pain and tension in muscles and tendons

Applications: massage, compresses, salve

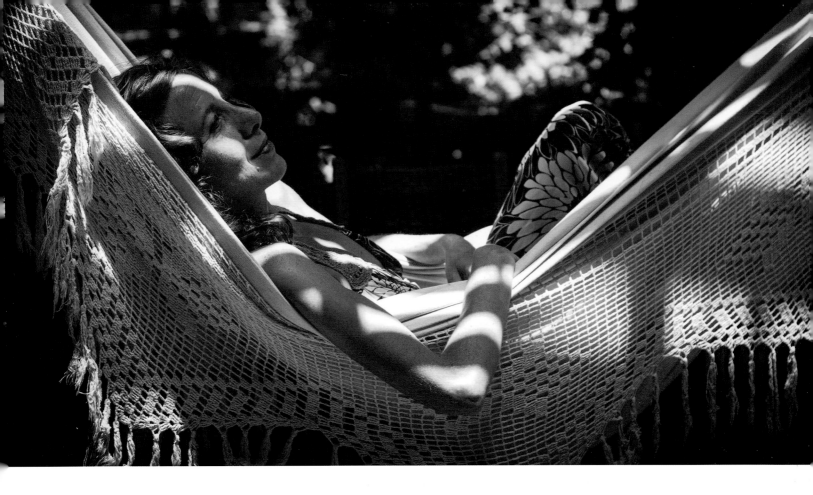

Cultivating Authentic Sensuality

Wear aromatic flowers in your hair.

Wear natural fabrics such as cashmere, cotton, silk, hemp, wool, linen, and alpaca.

Oil your skin with essential oils and jojoba or coconut oil when still wet from the shower.

Anoint pure perfume to all of your pulse points: on neck; behind ears; on wrists; behind knees; at ankles; on inner thighs; between your breasts.

Listen to soulful music.

Slowly and lovingly brush your hair with an essential oil.

Bathe in flower petals and essential oils.

Exercise and sweat. Healthy, strong, and calm is sexy.

Touch yourself slowly and lovingly to feel the softness of your skin all over your body.

Turn the lights down low. Light beeswax candles.

Practice self-breast massage. It's a beautiful act of self-love and a fun way to spend an afternoon.

Paint your toenails red.

Use feathers, leathers, and fruit in the bedroom. Use your imagination.

Throw out all of your old, tattered, and ugly underwear and replace it with something new, fresh, and lacy. Buy yourself one pair of exciting undies at least once a year. Invest in colored panties too, if only for the innocent joy of wearing funder-pants.

Wear high heels on occasion. Strut your stuff when you do, because you're the living embodiment of feminine power and charm.

Eat slowly. Chew each bite. Food is endlessly sexy. Don't let that opportunity go to waste by gulping it down without any thought.

Drink fine red wine and French champagne.

Give yourself a head massage and gently pull your hair.

Slowly move your hips in full circles. Start with your knees slightly bent. Move your hips side to side and then front to back. Move into making full circles in both directions. Watch yourself in the mirror to see where there's resistance to movement. There's power in those hips.

Engage your pelvic floor by pulling in the muscles you use to stop urine flow. Try to hold it at 30 percent for a longer time rather than 100 percent for less.

Use organic roses in cooking and rose water.

Smile. The divine expresses its joy through your smile, and you look pretty, too.

Pick wild flowers and arrange them in beautiful ways throughout your home.

Be quiet. We're able to sharpen our senses and become present in the quiet.

Lie naked in the sunshine. It feels really good.

Kiss flower petals and feel their soft and inviting petals kissing you back.

Eat oysters that are sustainably harvested from safe shores. Oysters are high in zinc. They boost testosterone and enhance your juicy power.

Dance to slow music, even by yourself.

Take a hula hoop, pole dance, or belly dance class to release your inner siren. She's aching to be freed and may be liberated by the experience.

Stand up straight with your shoulders back, stomach engaged, head held high, and chest open. Walk with poised determination. This is true sexy power.

Take deep breaths and relax your brow. Allow your teeth to separate slightly. Let your eyes rest in their sockets. Go down your entire body and allow every part, organ, and nerve to relax.

Kiss your lover for at least thirty seconds a day, deeply and with intent. There's a lot of information in a kiss.

Go commando-style by wearing no panties. It's a delicious little secret for you to keep.

Let chocolate melt in your mouth before slowly swallowing it.

Skinny-dip, preferably by moonlight.

Tell yourself positive affirmations about your body and beauty. You're only as beautiful as you believe you are.

Travel to an exotic destination. Feel the thrill of a new environment.

Practice winking and then try it out on a handsome stranger.

Light a fire in a fireplace or fire pit. Romance happens by flickering lights.

Buy yourself something scandalous and inappropriate, even if it's for your eyes only.

Practice gratitude.

Eat healthy, organic food.

Harvest your own spring water and sip it slowly in fancy glasses.

Laugh so hard that your insides joyfully hurt.

Look for the divine in everything.

Keep your heart as light as a feather. If it is heavier, you are losing the battle.

Do something kind for someone else. An open, loving heart might just be the most sensual thing of all.

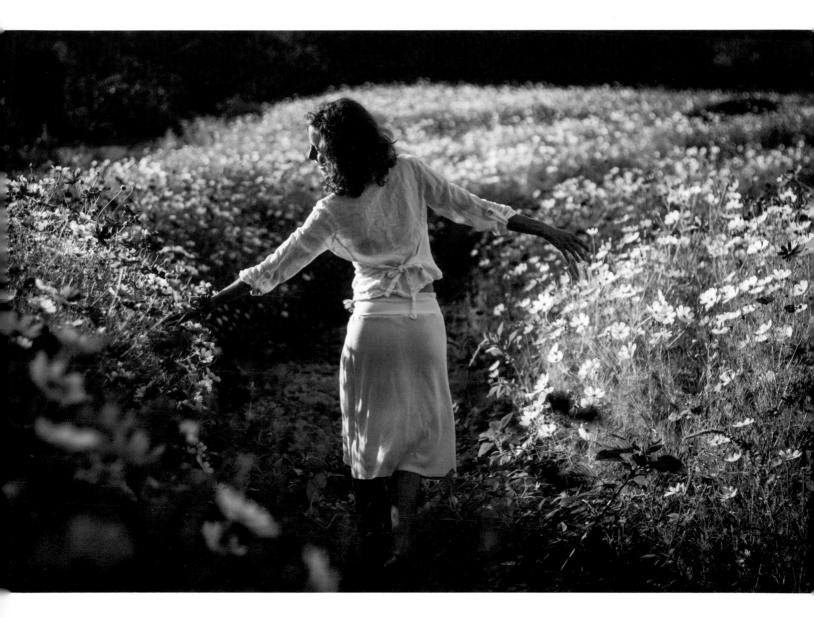

aromatherapy for sensual living *cultivating authentic sensuality*

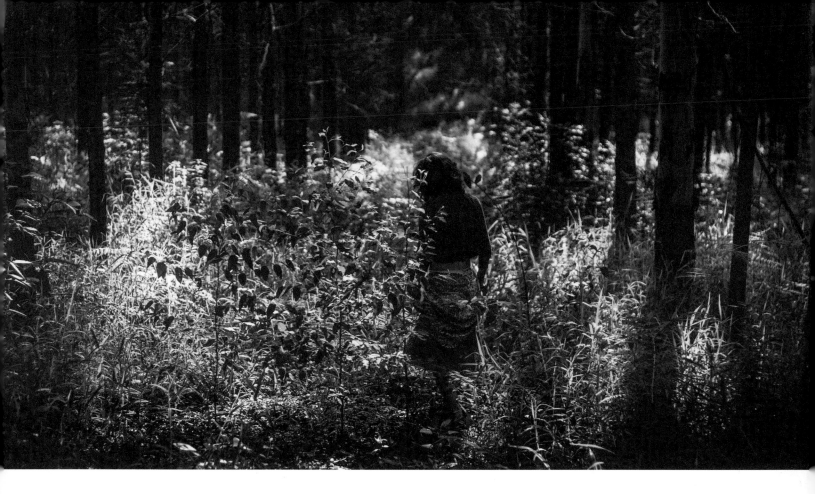

Be the Flower

"And the day came when the risk to stay tight in a bud was more painful than the risk to blossom."
– Anais Nin

Flowers are endlessly attractive and refined. By intimately acquainting your body with them, you take on their essence and become the flower. It is the quickest path to love.

Always smell good (with pure and natural essentials). Good things happen when you do. Don't miss an opportunity to broadcast your beauty, vitality, and love for the whole world to see. Be sure to have a couple of bottles on hand for an immediate aromatic enhancement. Aim to anoint yourself generously at least once a day as you would brush your teeth or hair. In doing so, you will open your heart to invite and receive more divine grace.

Shake the dew off your lily and invite flower power into your life. I dare you to gorge on nature's bounty; bathe in essential oils; feast on natural organic whole foods; celebrate health with natural medicines; drink spring water; plant a garden; and dig your feet in the dirt to connect to the earth. We get to reclaim a pure (and often repressed) aspect of ourselves. To become the flower, commune honestly

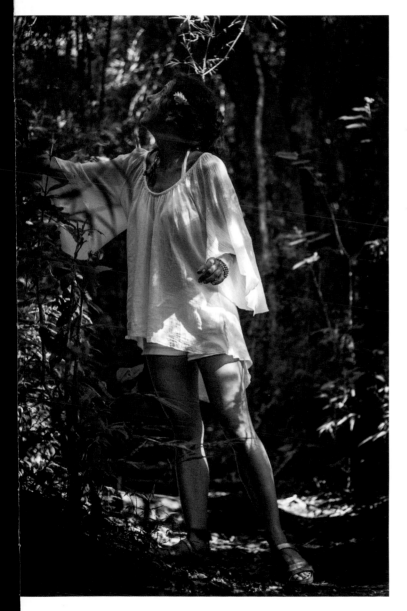

and authentically with the nature world every day. Be natural, naked, and claim your inherent beauty. It's your sexy power in action.

Please remember, in periods of deep sadness, know that joy hasn't abandoned you, because flowers are patiently holding it and waiting for your return.

Aroma is love never-ending.

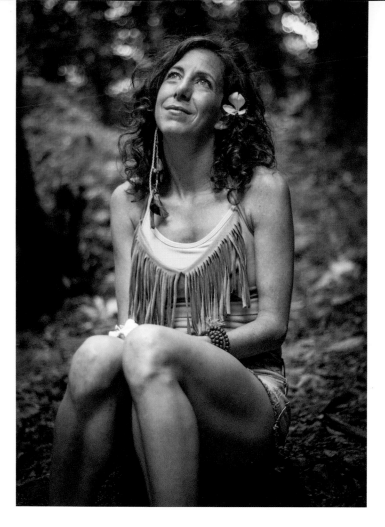

About the Author

Elana Millman started her passionate lifelong love affair with essential oils as a teenager and has used them every day for every aspect of life for twenty years. She trained extensively with Nadine Artemis of Living Libations and the Transformational Arts College in Toronto to refine her knowledge and create a unique way of understanding and using oils. She has taught workshops in Canada, Brazil, and Japan on erotics, exotics, euphorics, medicinal aromatherapy, essential oils for beauty, cleaning your home without chemicals, aromatherapy for women at every stage, and essential oils and the endocrine/chakra system.

Elana lives between Toronto, Canada and Rio de Janeiro, Brazil. In addition to being a holistic healer and aromatherapist, she's the co-founder of **pür frequency**, a line of CBD-infused aromatherapy products for beauty, health, and lifestyle. Visit www.purfrequency.com and www.thesensualliving.com for more details.

Elana started her writing career after graduating university when she worked as an international journalist in Europe, Asia, and the Caribbean. That experience inadvertently introduced her to the world of healing arts when she started receiving regular reflexology foot massages everywhere her job sent her. Not surprisingly, her little bottles of essential oils also supported her vitality and eased the stress associated with travel.

Elana is passionate about helping people understand the power of plants. She's dedicated to teaching how to empower health, healing, and sensuality with the use of essential oils.